Blacks in Medicine

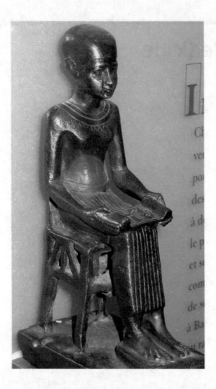

Statuette of Imhotep in the Louvre, Paris. (Image courtesy of Hu Totya CC 3.0) (By anonymous, CC BY-SA 3.0, https://commons.wikimedia.org/w/index.php?curid=657268)

Imhotep, son of mythical creator god Ptah, was born in Egypt about 3000 BCE. During his life, he was renowned as a philosopher, sage, scribe, poet, astronomer, chief lector priest, magician, and architect. He designed and constructed the first man-made stone structure, the Step Pyramid at Saqqara, part of the necropolis of the ancient Egyptian city of Memphis.

He was most famed for his skill as a physician and is generally considered the original author of the content of the *Edwin Smith Papyrus*, the oldest known surgical treatise on trauma (ca. 1600 BCE), which contains almost 100 anatomical terms and describes 48 injuries and their treatment. (Many historians believe that the text of the Smith papyrus was copied from a much older document originally written by Imhotep.) The first phrases of the Smith papyrus demonstrate that thousands of years before William Harvey, the ancient Egyptians directly associated the pulse with the heart, understanding its importance as the central organ of the body. In the papyrus, injuries are assessed with palpation, described and diagnosed rationally, with treatment, prognosis, and explanatory notes.

Imhotep was the first known physician to extract medicine from plants and is remembered for viewing disease and injury as naturally occurring, not as punishments inflicted by the gods, spirits, or curses. He was known as a medical demigod 100 years after his death and was elevated as a full deity by the Egyptians in c. 525 BCE, paving the way thousands of years before the arrival of the Greek/Roman god Asclepius and the Greek father of medicine, Hippocrates.

Richard Allen Williams

Blacks in Medicine

Clinical, Demographic, and Socioeconomic Correlations

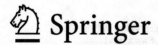

Richard Allen Williams
Encino, CA
USA

ISBN 978-3-030-41962-2   ISBN 978-3-030-41960-8   (eBook)
https://doi.org/10.1007/978-3-030-41960-8

This Springer imprint is published by the registered company Springer Nature Switzerland AG
The registered company address is: Gewerbestrasse 11, 6330 Cham, Switzerland

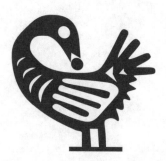

The symbol for the new book is the African Sankofa bird, a mythical animal depicted in the Akan (Adinkra) writing system as flying forward with its head turned backward. The egg in its mouth represents the "gems" or knowledge of the past upon which wisdom is based; it also signifies the generation to come that would benefit from that wisdom. This symbol may be associated with the Akan proverb, "se wo were fi na wasankofa a yenki," which means "it is not wrong to go back for what you have forgotten."

Book Theme

"Baraka Sasa," an old Swahili expression meaning "blessings now."

By ten things is the world created,
By wisdom and by understanding,
And by reason and by strength,
By rebuke and by might,
By righteousness and by judgment,
By loving kindness and by compassion.

–Talmud Higaga 12A

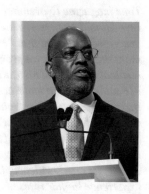

The sudden and unexpected passing of Bernard J. Tyson on November 10, 2019, at the age of 60 was a tragic loss not only for his family, friends, and colleagues but for the world of healthcare. As chairman and CEO of Kaiser Permanente, the giant HMO, he had taken corporate responsibility in healthcare delivery to a new level during his tenure at Kaiser's helm beginning in 2013. During this time, he presided over an increase in Kaiser's fortunes from 9.1 million members and an annual revenue of $53 billion in 2013 to 12.3 million members and revenue of $79.7 billion in 2018. In addition, he remained steadfastly within the Affordable Care Act (ObamaCare) as a member of the exchanges in California at a time when other major insurers bailed out in 2017. I had the opportunity to speak with him about how to deal with healthcare deficiencies and disparities suffered by blacks and other minorities when I invited him to give the keynote speech at the

National Medical Association Colloquium in Los Angeles in March 2016. That is when I learned of his plan to build a new medical school in Pasadena, California, that would focus on recruiting disadvantaged underrepresented minority students and providing tuition-free medical education for them. True to his word, Kaiser is set to open its medical school in Pasadena in 2020, and tuition will be waived for the first five classes. (One might say that this is truly "putting your money where your mouth is.")

Six days before he died, Tyson published an article in Time magazine (November 4, 2019) titled "Where You Live Should Not Determine Your Healthcare." In it, he described his belief that "Health is about so much more than the care we provide at a hospital or medical office." He also stated that "An individual's ZIP code can be a more accurate driver of health than their genetic code," an opinion also articulated in Chap. 9 of this book. What he was stressing was his belief in the importance of the socioeconomics of health and its impact on communities. In the Time article, he cited evidence that select neighborhoods experience higher rates of certain diseases and went on to show how healthcare organizations such as Kaiser can participate in solving the multitude of problems facing impacted communities. In line with this philosophy, he further stated that "It is time for us to engage in the fight for health beyond our walls." and presented Kaiser's approach to this by launching a social health network which he called "Thrive Local" in which their technology partner Unite Us is integrated into Kaiser's electronic health record system, which allows healthcare workers to refer clients who are in need of special services directly to community organizations and social service agencies that can help them. And stepping up to the plate of financial need again, Kaiser made an impact investment of $200 million last year to address homelessness and housing affordability.

It should be obvious, therefore, that Bernard J. Tyson was a man who deserves to have a book dealing with healthcare issues facing vulnerable populations dedicated to him. He has not only talked the talk—he also walked the walk. I consider him a true hero in the struggle against healthcare disparities. A giant has fallen, but hopefully his example and the lessons he taught us will be perpetuated and will help us to realize the motto that Tyson authored in 2004 as a senior vice president and that Kaiser Permanente still uses today—"thrive."

Richard Allen Williams, MD

Foreword

The farther backward you can look, the farther forward you can see.

This statement, attributed to Sir Winston Churchill, epitomizes the importance of recognizing the past as a prologue to the future, which is a tenet that Dr. Richard Allen Williams has observed in writing *Blacks in Medicine*. This book, his ninth volume contributed to the medical literature, is a sweeping and comprehensive exposition that covers the broad field of clinical medicine, that delves into the demographic aspects of healthcare delivery, and that intermixes a societal component consisting of the socioeconomics of health, all superimposed on a historical background dating back 5000 years to Imhotep, the Egyptian/Nubian who was the first doctor known to the world, and ranging forward over the centuries and millennia to the present time. I would conjecture that such a complex interplay of multiple factors incorporating numerous dimensions into a single book is a rarity in medical writing, and it is indicative of the fact that Dr. Williams, the sole author, has a gift for this type of endeavor. However, knowing him as I do, I would not expect anything less based on his almost encyclopedic knowledge of all of the discrete ingredients that he has placed into the mix, as well as the clinical, educational, and institutional experience that he has gained over the past 50 years.

Those ingredients form the substance of the book's main purpose, which is to focus attention on the long-running crisis in healthcare delivery faced every day by 40 million African Americans, who are constantly besieged by medical problems that threaten their survival as a race. It leads off with a description and an analysis of some of the principal threats that are delivered up to the black population as examples of healthcare disparities, thus carrying on the theme of inequities in health status and healthcare delivery that was initially articulated in Dr. Williams's iconic book *Textbook of Black-Related Diseases* (1975) (now in the Smithsonian Institution), continued with the *Report of the Secretary's Task Force on Black & Minority Health* (1985) (also known as the Heckler Report), and punctuated with the Institute of Medicine (IOM) Report in the groundbreaking book *Unequal Treatment: Confronting Racial and Ethnic Disparities in Health Care* (2002), which set the tone for how we view healthcare disparities. The historical component is invoked early on, and repeated references to slavery as the root cause of the deficient and inequitable healthcare system are made, as emphatically and expertly detailed by Byrd and Clayton in their blockbuster work, *An American Health*

Dilemma: A Medical History of African Americans and the Problem of Race: Beginnings to 1900 (2000). The perspective of the African American medical practitioner is also in focus as an integral part of the black experience in medicine. This is a topic that I have written about in my book, *Seeing Patients: Unconscious Bias in Health Care* (2011), in which the unique view of medicine as seen through the eyes of a black doctor is presented; it contains some explanation of how healthcare disparities occur and what can be done to prevent them.

Historical details about African American doctors and our trials and tribulations in attempting to establish a healthcare capability of our own are very richly described in *Blacks in Medicine*, and the legacy of those physicians who sacrificed so much in order to do this is documented with a recognition of some of the outstanding blacks in the medical history of the United States. Although this has been attempted in several books and papers in the past, such as in the late Dr. Claude Organ's magnificent two-volume book, *A Century of Black Surgeons* (1987), the descriptions have been fragmentary. Although Dr. Williams recognizes that he cannot include everyone who deserves such recognition, he has done a commendable job in highlighting many who have worked in the trenches, caring for indigent black patients and leading the struggle for justice in healthcare delivery and education without adequate return or sufficient reward for so long. The struggle to establish black medical schools and hospitals for the education and treatment of African Americans is explored as a part of the historical exposition.

Nothing in the current context of healthcare delivery is more impactful than the issue of healthcare reform and all of the political implications associated with it. Accordingly, this book continues the examination of that subject that Dr. Williams wrote extensively about in his highly regarded book, *Healthcare Disparities at the Crossroads with Healthcare Reform* (Springer, 2011). It is fitting that the discussion of this subject is open-ended, because the nation is still attempting to determine the most appropriate healthcare system to adopt. Thus, the book has a great deal of current relevance regarding the political scene, especially as this issue affects African Americans.

After entering into a discourse on the current health status of blacks, including their longevity, some surprising statistics and trends are revealed that are emblematic of the unique nature of disease affecting the black population. This is particularly significant since this information can inform our healthcare system about whether the medical treatment of African Americans is headed in the right direction, and it also suggests what changes may be needed to alter the course. This could be critical in the long term.

Finally, the book winds up with a chapter on the socioeconomic determinants of health, which Dr. Williams declares is a more important issue than access to care. This has to do primarily with the factors that impact us in our neighborhoods and communities of risk, such as the environment, housing, poverty, clean water, food resources, income, and access to medical resources. This is the most forward-looking part of the book, and it encompasses the overarching issue that he strongly feels holds the greatest promise for eliminating disparities and for making a real impact on the healthcare crisis that we have endured as a race for the past 400 years since American slavery began in 1619. Dr. Williams's analysis is deeply insightful and contains wisdom that is crucial to the interests and survival of African American patients.

The legendary late poet and writer, Maya Angelou, wrote a poignant poem that speaks to the horrible conditions that have been imposed upon blacks for centuries and also to the resiliency, determination, and strength that black people have demonstrated in surviving those oppressive conditions. Below is an excerpt.

Out of the huts of history's shame
I rise
Up from a past that's rooted in pain
I rise
I'm a black ocean, leaping and wide,
Welling and swelling I bear in the tide.

Leaving behind nights of terror and fear
I rise
Into a daybreak that's wondrously clear
I rise
Bringing the gifts that my ancestors gave,
I am the dream and the hope of the slave.
I rise
I rise
I rise.

And like the air, whose indomitable spirit was extolled in this poem, African American people will continue to rise despite repeatedly being knocked down and run over time and time again. This splendid book, *Blacks in Medicine*, will provide some of the information that we need to survive and prevail in an increasingly hostile environment. It is recommended reading for everyone, not only for African American families involved with healthcare but especially for medical caregivers engaged in the contemporary healthcare industry.

Augustus A. White, III, MD, PhD
Ellen and Melvin Gordon Distinguished Professor of Medical Education
Former Advisory Dean, Oliver Wendell Holmes Society
Professor of Orthopaedic Surgery
Orthopaedic Surgeon-in-Chief Emeritus, Beth Israel Hospital
Harvard Medical School
Boston, Massachusetts

Preface

The subject of health problems in blacks is not well known and has not been adequately researched. This deficiency in our knowledge base has had serious medical consequences, such as incorrect treatment of certain diseases and lack of information regarding the fact that blacks may have different illness characteristics than whites. I first called attention to this situation in the *Textbook of Black-Related Diseases*, which I authored in 1975. Although that publication was successful in shedding light on the fact that blacks possess special medical circumstances and may have different healthcare needs, it did not explore the complete context of these problems over the course of history. Unless it is known how certain medical problems originate and evolve over time, it's impossible to fully comprehend the impact that this problem may have on a group of people. Solutions to those problems also depend in part on that relationship.

What is also implied here is that the historical context in which medical problems occur can influence their clinical expression. For example, poor medical treatment of blacks in the South for conditions such as tuberculosis led to the development of chronicity and resistance as well as endemic spread of this disease. This was documented among black mill workers in the twentieth-century South. It was not until public health measures were instituted that this deadly situation was improved. Another example is the transmission of infectious diseases such as measles from one society where it prevailed to another where no immunity existed. This occurred in several instances in history, including the transmission of measles to the Hawaiian Islands in the seventeenth century that virtually wiped out the indigenous native Hawaiian population and to Africa in the fifteenth century. Unless medical conditions are viewed in the temporal, demographic, and socioeconomic milieu in which they occur, the complete picture of how and why they affect certain groups of people such as blacks in a fashion that is different from the usual way will not be completely understood. Although it has been well established that blacks and whites may experience disease differently, the impact of factors such as time, environment, and poverty must be analyzed along with the clinical presentation of illness; otherwise, attempts to treat the condition successfully may fail, and prevention of similar cases among others in that same group may not be possible.

This small book is being written to answer some questions as to why there has been a pattern of poor and deficient health status among blacks throughout their history. It is not sufficient to blame everything on slavery; that theory is too simplistic to explain all of the peculiarities of diseases of blacks. Racism, which has been a pervasive and nefarious social attitude in the United States and throughout the world throughout recorded history, has been documented repeatedly, but it is not the entire reason for the phenomenon either. Recently, we have learned to appreciate the impact of what are called the socioeconomic (or social) determinants of health, and these factors are examined in the book as to how they influence and shape the expression of illness in blacks as well as the delivery of healthcare. This is a new and very essential paradigm in our approach to the question of how to improve healthcare delivery for blacks.

Another dimension that this book contains is an analysis of the medical education system in the United States and how its deficiencies affect black health. This pertains to the inadequate education of blacks throughout our history and the insufficient production of African American medical professionals that has handicapped our desire to be able to treat and to heal ourselves. We have found ourselves in a most peculiar and very precarious situation, in which black citizens have been poorly treated by the predominantly white medical system, while at the same time, we have been denied the means of taking care of ourselves. Black civil rights activist Fannie Lou Hamer declared that "we're sick and tired of being sick and tired"; underlying that poignant expression was a frustration with a healthcare system that does not deliver on its promise to provide excellent treatment for all, regardless of race and ethnicity.

Certainly, it is important to highlight the efforts and contributions of black doctors and other healthcare professionals in order to paint a better picture of how blacks have been a part of the medical equation. These individuals, who should be regarded as nothing less than heroes in our society, have been accorded little recognition in our standard medical history texts and in fact have been excluded from mainstream medicine for most of our history. They should be lauded and elevated to their proper places in the pantheon of medical heroes, and their clinical exploits should be broadly appreciated by students and practitioners of medicine. One of the purposes of this book is to attempt to do just that.

There have been several books that have documented the role of blacks in medical history, and although that has been an important function, that is not the main purpose of this one. The principal wish is to link clinical experiences that blacks have had with the surrounding and perhaps causative factors that relate to their poor health status compared to that of whites. In addition, there is an attempt to use the information supplied to suggest preventive measures that might keep history from repeating itself to the continued detriment of our black citizens. In other words, it is an effort to use the examples of history as lessons that may be employed to provide a transition to a new era in which these historical elements become tools that help to improve black health status and to eliminate healthcare disparities, which is dealt with in the last part of the book in conjunction with an analysis of the Affordable Care Act. Thus, the circle of literary exposition going from ancient origins of the healthcare problems of blacks to the present-day efforts to achieve equity in healthcare delivery will have been completed, carrying out my intentions proclaimed in two of my previous books, *Eliminating Healthcare Disparities in America: Beyond the IOM Report* (Humana, 2007) and *Healthcare Disparities at the Crossroads with Healthcare Reform* (Springer, 2011). It should be understood that this is not an attempt to provide all of the answers to the question of why blacks suffer from deficient health status; rather, it intends to provoke thought about the origins of those problems and how they may be linked to factors that connote a certain sickness in our society.

This is the last of nine books that I have authored on the general subject of healthcare disparities and the need for greater understanding of the health problems of minority populations and of blacks in particular. I hope that I have provided some information to give incentive to younger generations of health equity activists, whom I challenge with the question: *What will you do with it?*

Encino, CA, USA   Richard Allen Williams, MD, FACC, FAHA, FACP

Acknowledgments

Anyone who has ever attempted to write a book knows that it involves more than one person, even if there is only a single author. This book is an example of that dictum. I would like to express my deep gratitude to my colleagues, friends, students, and mentees who voluntarily provided significant input and contributed in various ways to its completion. The main helpers were Darlene Parker-Kelly; Winston Price, MD; Genita Evangelista Johnson; Tselane Gardner; Yasmine Griffiths; Dimeji Williams; Dr. Sylvia Drew Ivie; Erin Johnson; Cassandra McCullough; Jeryl Bryant; Tierra Dillenburg; Yvette Lee; Rachel Williams; and Katrese Phelps-McCullum. There were others who helped but are too numerous to name.

I also want to recognize the outstanding guidance and assistance given to me by my developmental editor, Katherine Kreilkamp, who urged me on for 3 difficult years to complete the book.

Richard Allen Williams, MD

Contents

About the Author

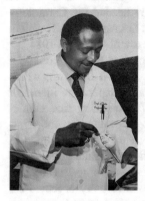

Dr. Richard Allen Williams was impacted by healthcare disparities from birth when he was delivered by a midwife at home in the ghetto of Wilmington, Delaware, just as his seven older siblings had been, because his parents could not afford hospital care. When he was a toddler, he almost died from severe pneumonia that he contracted from living in substandard housing under wintry conditions. However, he was able literally to weather the storm and not only to survive but also to thrive. Attending all-black schools in segregated Wilmington from kindergarten through 12th grade, he graduated at the top of his class and won a full scholarship to Harvard in 1953 as the first black student from Delaware to matriculate there. His Harvard class of 1957, which celebrated its 60th anniversary in 2017, was the first to have integrated dormitories and dining facilities. However, the private fraternities, called eating clubs, were closed to him. He graduated with honors and went on to graduate from medical school at the State University of New York Downstate Medical Center, which bestowed an Honorary Doctor of Humane Letters degree upon him last year at Carnegie Hall. He subsequently became the first African American intern at the University of California, San Francisco Medical Center and later became the first black postgraduate fellow (Cardiology) at Brigham and Women's Hospital and Harvard Medical School.

While at the Brigham, he established a groundbreaking program called the Central Recruitment Council in collaboration with Harvard Medical School Dean Dr. Robert H. Ebert, which was successful in recruiting black students and postgraduate trainees (interns, residents, and fellows) for the first time in Harvard's storied history. He was given a Lifetime Achievement Award for this pivotal accomplishment, which changed the face of diversity at Harvard. He later joined the Harvard Medical School Faculty as an instructor and junior associate in Medicine, following which he accepted an appointment at the new Dr. Martin Luther King, Jr. Community Hospital in Watts, California, as the inaugural assistant medical director in 1972. It was there that he succeeded in securing a $2.7 million grant from NIH to establish the King-Drew Sickle Cell Center, one of the first in the nation, of which he became the director. He moved to UCLA in 1974 and eventually headed the Cardiology Department at the UCLA-West Los Angeles VA Hospital. He was promoted to full professor at UCLA in 1984.

In 1975, McGraw-Hill published his first book, the pioneering *Textbook of Black-Related Diseases*, which was a presentation on how blacks experience illness. It emphasized the importance of recognizing race, ethnicity, and culture in the diagnosis, evaluation, and treatment of patients and the need to collect health data according to the patient's racial and ethnic designation, which the federal government and other healthcare entities now do. His first book was recently accepted for inclusion in the National Museum of African American History and Culture of the Smithsonian Institution, the first medical book written by a black physician to be so honored. He also edited several other books, including *Humane Medicine*, Vols. I and II (1999, 2001); *The Athlete and Heart Disease: Diagnosis, Evaluation & Management* (1999); *Eliminating Healthcare Disparities in America: Beyond the IOM Report* (2007); *The Heart of The Matter* (2008); and *Healthcare Disparities at the Crossroads with Healthcare Reform* (2011).

He was the Founder of the Association of Black Cardiologists (ABC) in 1974 and of the Minority Health Institute (1985). In 2016, he was elected President of the National Medical Association. He has received many honors, awards, and honorary degrees and was inducted into Fellowships of the American College of Cardiology (FACC), the American Heart Association (FAHA), and the American College of Physicians (FACP). In 2014, he was the first black physician to receive the LifeSaver Award from the American Heart Association. In 2019, he received both the inaugural Distinguished Award for Diversity and Inclusion from the American College of

Cardiology and the inaugural Excellence in Medicine Humanitarian Award from the American Medical Association Foundation in recognition of his 50 years of accomplishments and dedication to eliminating healthcare disparities. More recently, he received the iconic John P. McGovern Compleat Physician Award from the Houston Academy of Medicine, following a tradition established by Osler, Cooley, and DeBakey.

Five Diseases That Are Devastating the African American Population

1

Sickle Cell Disease

Historical Background and Pathophysiology

Some authorities consider sickle cell anemia the "poster child" of diseases primarily affecting blacks, or what the author calls black-related diseases, as described in 1975 in the *Textbook of Black-Related Diseases* [1].

Sickle cell disease (SCD) consists of several related blood dyscrasias that are linked by a disorder of hemoglobin and are therefore called hemoglobinopathies. They include homozygous hemoglobin S disease (HbSS), sickle hemoglobin C disease (HbSC), and several genotypes of sickle beta-thalassemia as well as other genetic subtypes that are due to compound heterozygosity for the HbS gene and other variants of hemoglobin, including HbC, HbE, and HbD. Sickle cell anemia, the most prominent of these disorders, was identified by James B. Herrick in 1910 [2]. Dr. Herrick was the attending physician for intern Ernest Irons who had a black patient from Grenada who was severely anemic. On examining the patient's blood smear, Dr. Herrick noted what he called sickle-shaped red blood cells (Figs. 1.1 and 1.2). (They were so-called because their shape looked like the sickle that was used to cut sugar cane.) His description of the disease was known for many years as *Herrick's syndrome*, later known as sickle cell syndrome, and eventually as sickle cell anemia. The full significance of the disorder was not appreciated until Dr. Linus Pauling described the molecular abnormality and pathophysiology of SCD in 1949 [3]. Pauling and his team found that the disease was caused by a missense mutation on the beta globin gene of normal hemoglobin (HbA) in which the amino acid glutamic acid was substituted for the amino acid valine (Fig. 1.3) [4].

This leads to deoxygenation and polymerization of the hemoglobin molecule and the formation of hemoglobin S (HbS). Consequently, the red blood cells are deformed, and the misshapen cells are unable to navigate smoothly through the blood vessels of the body, thus causing obstructions in the various organs (Fig. 1.4).

© Springer Nature Switzerland AG 2020

R. A. Williams, *Blacks in Medicine*, https://doi.org/10.1007/978-3-030-41960-8_1

Fig. 1.1 Sickle cells in human blood; both normal red blood cells and sickle-shaped cells are present. (Courtesy of Dr. Graham Beards—own work, CC BY-SA 3.0, https://commons. wikimedia.org/w/index. php?curid=18421017)

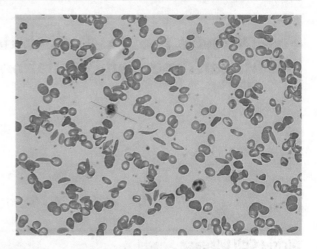

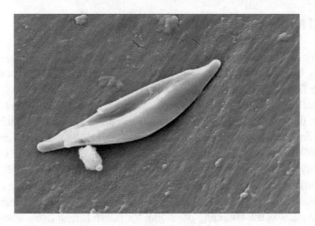

Fig. 1.2 Electron microscopic image of a sickled erythrocyte found in the blood of an 18-year-old female patient with sickle cell anemia (HbSS). (Centers for Disease Control and Prevention Public Health Image Library (PHIL)/Sickle Cell Foundation of Georgia: Jackie George, Beverly Sinclair. Photograph credit: Janice Haney Carr. https://phil.cdc.gov/Details. aspx?pid=11688#modalIdString_imgURL1)

Increased hemolysis also occurs, leading to hemolytic anemia and release of free iron into the blood. These pathological changes result in the myriad symptoms of sickle cell anemia, the worst of which are the pain crises. These are episodes of vascular occlusion caused by erythrocyte and leukocyte adhesion to the endothelium. Blood flow to vital organs is impaired, leading to tissue ischemia and excruciating pain throughout the body [5, 6]. Virtually all patients with sickle cell anemia are in danger of death at an early age due to the ravages of the disease, with life expectancy reduced by about 30 years (Fig. 1.5) [7].

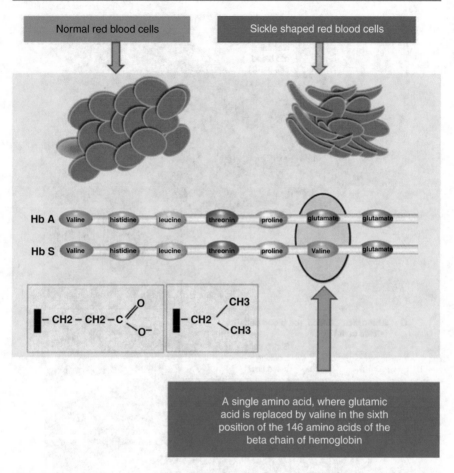

Fig. 1.3 Diagram showing the change of a single amino acid, in which glutamic acid is replaced by valine in the sixth position of the 146 amino acids of the beta chain of hemoglobin. This leads to the formation of hemoglobin S and a change of the normal red blood cells to sickle-shaped red blood cells. (From Al-Salem [4], with permission)

Epidemiology

Sickle cell disease is the most common monogenic disease in the world [8]. It is estimated that 300,000 babies are born each year with the homozygous form of the disease, sickle cell anemia. Most of these births occur in Nigeria, the Democratic Republic of the Congo, and India. The disease is also very prevalent in sub-Saharan Africa, the Mediterranean basin, and the Middle East. In the United States, the vast majority of the victims are black, numbering an estimated 100,000 [7, 9–11] (Figs. 1.6 and 1.7). According to the US Department of Health and Human Services Office of

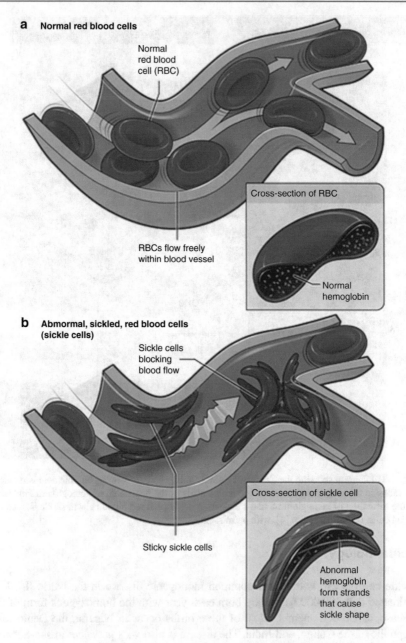

Fig. 1.4 Pathophysiology of sickle cell anemia in which abnormal sickle-shaped red blood cells obstruct normal blood flow, causing ischemia and pain crises. (Panel **a**) shows normal red blood cells flowing freely through veins. The inset shows a cross section of a normal red blood cell with normal hemoglobin. (Panel **b**) shows abnormal, sickled red blood cells sticking at the branching point in a vein. The inset image shows a cross section of a sickle cell with long polymerized sickle hemoglobin (HbS) strands stretching and distorting the cell shape to look like a crescent. (Courtesy of the National Heart, Lung, and Blood Institute [NHLBI] http://www.nhlbi.nih.gov/health/health-topics/topics/sca/, Public Domain, https://commons.wikimedia.org/w/index.php?curid=19198765)

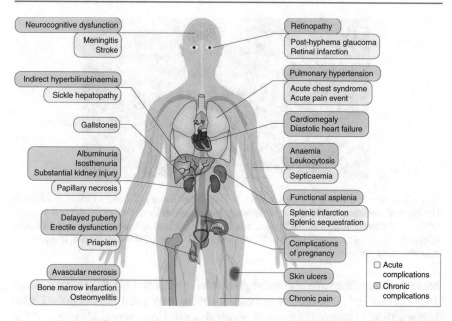

Fig. 1.5 Sickle cell disease clinical complications. Pain is the most common acute complication. As individuals with SCD age, chronic complications produce organ dysfunction that can contribute to earlier death. There are numerous complications in pregnancy. (From Kato et al. [7], with permission from Springer Nature)

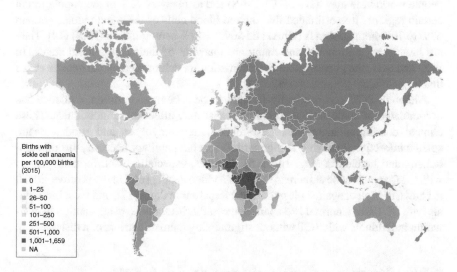

Fig. 1.6 Map of the estimated numbers of births with sickle cell anemia. Per 100,000 births per country in 2015. Estimates are derived from prevalence data published in Piel et al. [10]. Birth data for 2015–2020 were extracted from the 2017 Revision of the United Nations World Population database. (From Kato et al. [7], with permission from Springer Nature)

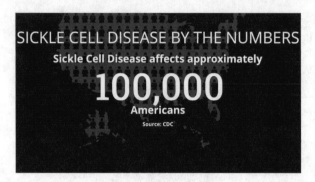

Fig. 1.7 According to the US Department of Health and Human Services Office of Minority Health, there are about 100,000 people currently living with sickle cell disease;, the vast majority of them are African American. SCD occurs in 1 out 365 African American births, 1 in 13 babies (Courtesy US Department of Health and Human Services Office of Minority Health. https://www.minorityhealth.hhs.gov/sicklecell/)

Minority Health (https://www.minorityhealth.hhs.gov/sicklecell), SCD occurs among 1 out of every 365 black or African American births, only 1 in 4 patients in the United States with SCD receive the standard of care described in current guidelines, and 1 in 13 black or African American babies is born with sickle cell trait.

About 8–10% of the African American population is affected by sickle cell trait (SCT), the heterozygous state of the sickle hemoglobin beta globin gene that is the carrier state of SCD, compared with 1% of whites [12, 13]. Up to 300 million people worldwide may have SCT (HbAS) and as many as 25% of the population in certain regions. It is estimated that the red blood cells of these individuals contain 60% to 70% hemoglobin A (HbA) and 30% to 40% hemoglobin S (HbS) [14]. They are largely asymptomatic, and many are unaware of their hemoglobin status. In SCD and SCT, the phenotypical characteristics are determined by the genetic status that an individual possesses (Fig. 1.8).

Although SCT was originally thought to be a benign condition, evidence has accumulated of some serious morbidities that may affect these individuals. These clinical conditions include exercise-related rhabdomyolysis and sudden death, splenic infarction occurring at high altitudes, renal papillary necrosis, thromboembolism, and hematuria (Fig. 1.9) [15]. Athletes, especially black football players with SCT, appear to be at increased risk of sudden death [16]. On the positive side, it is known to protect against plasmodium falciparum malaria [17], and most individuals with SCT live a normal life-span. Some authorities advise using caution in evaluating individuals with SCT without stigmatizing them as carriers of a disease [18].

Clinical, Therapeutic, and Healthcare Aspects in Sickle Cell Disease

An increased focus on SCD began in the 1920s when Dr. Lemuel Diggs, a pathologist in Memphis, Tennessee, noted a malaria-like illness in his area, which on pathological inspection turned out to be sickle cell anemia. It received some attention as a

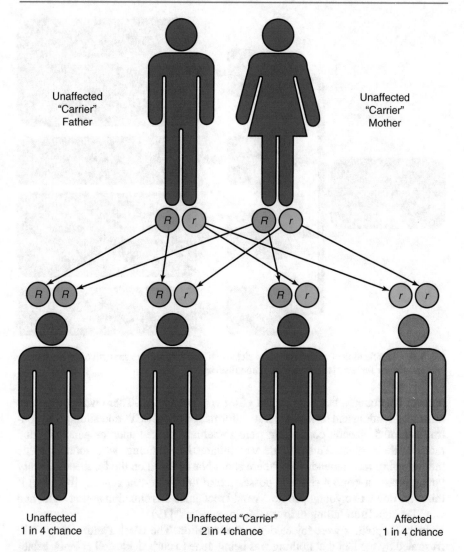

Fig. 1.8 Sickle cell disease is inherited in the autosomal recessive pattern. (Courtesy of Cburnett—own work in Inkscape, CC BY-SA 3.0, https://commons.wikimedia.org/w/index. php?curid=1840082)

medical curiosity through the next two decades, but its significance as a deadly disease of the blood that principally affected blacks was still not fully appreciated until Pauling described the molecular abnormalities that are characteristic of the illness in 1949. After that point, there was a surge of interest that carried through for two more decades and then waned. During that time, no specific therapy was developed for the victims except for symptomatic treatment. Societal pressure was applied by groups such as the Black Panthers about the fact that this disease that primarily affected blacks was essentially being ignored. The Black Panthers tried to take matters into their own hands by organizing public screening programs in various

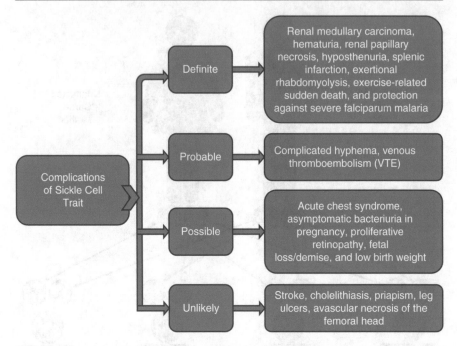

Fig. 1.9 Classification of complications of sickle cell trait according to strength of reported associations. (From Tantawy [15], with permission Elsevier)

parts of the country, but their valiant effort was insufficient. There was widespread misunderstanding and lack of accurate information about SCD, and attempts to control it through genetic counseling were sometimes looked upon as genocidal and racist in their intent. This attitude was inflamed by Pauling, who actually made the following recommendation: "there should be tattooed on the forehead of every young person a symbol showing possession of the sickle-cell gene…. [because] if this were done, two young people…would recognize this situation at first sight, and would refrain from falling in love with one another" [19].

In 1971, politics were injected into the situation. The Black Panther Party, still frustrated by the fact that nothing was being done to curb sickle cell anemia, established the Sickle Cell Anemia Research Foundation and conducted screening programs in several American cities. Not by coincidence, President Richard Nixon, apparently sensing the concerns of the public, voiced an interest in increasing funding for diagnosis, prevention, treatment, and counseling for SCD; he eventually signed the *National Sickle Cell Anemia Control Act of 1972* (Public law no. 92–294). Funds were made available through the National Institutes of Health (NIH) for the establishment of sickle cell clinics and centers around the country.

The author organized a grant proposal and submitted it to the NIH. It competed successfully for funding, garnering $2.74 million to establish the King-Drew Sickle Cell Center at the new Dr. Martin Luther King, Jr. Hospital in Watts, a private, nonprofit, safety-net hospital serving 1.3 million residents in South Los Angeles,

California. Dr. David Satcher, a future US Surgeon General, collaborated on that proposal and in the operation of the King-Drew Sickle Cell Center, which the author directed. Opening in 1972, it was one of the first in the nation. The late Roland B. Scott, Chief of Pediatrics at Howard University School of Medicine, also received a grant from the NIH and opened a sickle cell anemia center in the same year, as did the University of Southern California Sickle Cell Center operating under Drs. Darleen Powars, Julian Haywood, and Cage Johnson in Los Angeles. The King-Drew Sickle Cell Center closed years ago, but the new MLK Jr. Outpatient Center for Adults with SCD opened in 2016 in response to the great need in southern California (http://www.scdfc.org/scd-clinic-at-mlk.html_).

Meanwhile, research on genetic disorders such as cystic fibrosis, which mainly affects whites, has clearly outpaced research and efforts to find effective treatment and a cure for SCD, which has a much higher prevalence among the American population. One study comparing the two diseases indicated gross disparities between them. Sickle cell disease, which is three times more prevalent than cystic fibrosis (100,000 vs. 30,000), received much less funding support from NIH and from foundations [20].

We confirmed widely disparate NIH and national foundation funding per individual affected by SCD and cystic fibrosis. Research productivity as measured by articles indexed in PubMed, new clinical trials, and new drug approvals were substantially higher for cystic fibrosis, despite similar severity to SCD and many fewer affected individuals in the U.S.....

Funding per affected individual was 7.6 (2010) to 11.4-fold (2011) greater for cystic fibrosis than SCD and included a 3.5-fold higher NIH funding and 370 (2010) to 440 fold (2011) higher national foundation funding. NIH career development awards were similar for the two diseases despite nearly 3-fold more individuals affected by SCD. There were nearly twice as many publications and slightly more new listings of clinical trials for cystic fibrosis. No drugs were approved between 2010 and July 2013 for the treatment of SCD compared with 5 for cystic fibrosis [20].

This indicates a blatant disparity between the attention given to SCD, which primarily affects blacks, and cystic fibrosis, which mainly affects whites. Although both of these deadly diseases need adequate research and funding, there should be equity in the distribution of available resources.

Beginning in the 1970s, the treatment of SCD improved because of the introduction of hydroxyurea, which was not a panacea by any means but which did decrease the frequency of pain crises, primarily by increasing the levels of fetal hemoglobin (HbF) in the red blood cells of SCD patients, thus decreasing polymerization of HbS. Until very recently, hydroxyurea was the only drug approved by the US Food and Drug Administration (FDA) for the treatment of SCD [21].

Another key development was the introduction of antibiotics, especially penicillin, to treat infections such as pneumonia that often plagues SCD patients and is often the cause of death. Penicillin prophylaxis in children has been extremely impactful when administered as early as 2 months of age up to age 5, leading to a huge reduction in the infection rate and the death rate [22]. The beneficial results of the use of these two interventions, hydroxyurea and antibiotics, are seen in Fig. 1.10.

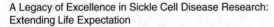

A Legacy of Excellence in Sickle Cell Disease Research:
Extending Life Expectation

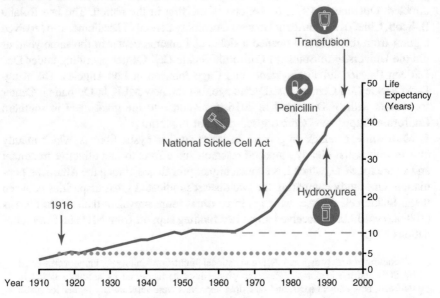

Fig. 1.10 Political and therapeutic interventions have led to increases in life expectancy for expectancy for patients with sickle cell disease (Courtesy of the National Heart, Lung, and Blood Institute [NHLBI] https://www.nhlbi.nih.gov/sites/default/files/inline-images/scd_bending-the-curve.jpg)

The politicization of the management of SCD, as alluded to above, has affected the clinical outcomes of efforts to prevent and treat the disease. Although there have been advances in supportive care and an increase in life expectancy in recent years—mainly due to antibiotic prophylaxis and treatment—a disparity in the extent of scientific attention given still exists between SCD and other genetic disorders. However, the development of new drugs for treatment of SCD is showing some signs of progress. Endari® (L-glutamine oral powder) recently won FDA approval for the treatment of complications and is the first drug for SCD to receive approval in the last 20 years. It is indicated for the treatment of SCD in adult and pediatric patients 5 years and older. Credit should be given to Yutaka Niihara (David Geffen School of Medicine at UCLA, Emmaus Life Sciences, Torrance CA, USA), who persisted for 25 years in developing the drug [23]. A recent phase III study of L-glutamine by Niihara showed "among children and adults with sickle cell anemia, the median number of pain crises over 48 weeks was lower among those who received oral therapy with l-glutamine, administered alone or with hydroxyurea, than among those who received placebo, with or without hydroxyurea (funded by Emmaus Medical; ClinicalTrials.gov number, NCT01179217)" [24]. Other drugs in phase II and III studies include crizanlizumab (Adakveo®) (SEG 101), an once-a-month intravenous monoclonal antibody against the adhesion molecule p-selectin that has shown promise in decreasing pain crises and complications such as the acute chest syndrome by limiting the adhesion of sickle erythrocytes to the endothelium of blood vessels [25], and voxelotor (Oxbryta™) developed by Global Blood Therapeutics (South San Francisco CA), largely due to the tireless efforts of Ted Love, MD. In September 2019 the FDA accepted for filing the company's New Drug Application seeking accelerated approval for the drug, an oral, once-daily therapy in development for the treatment of SCD. If approved, voxelotor would be the first therapy available to patients that targets hemoglobin polymerization, the root cause of SCD damage. A few other drugs are in the developmental pipeline [26]. Vichinsky and the HOPE trial investigators demonstrated that an HbS polymerization inhibitor has the potential to modify SCD by increasing hemoglobin levels and decreasing hemolysis [27]. In addition, significant reduction is now seen in serious complications such as primary stroke prevention via the use of frequent blood transfusions and transcranial Doppler screening [28].

Although no "magic bullet" has yet been invented to cure SCD without causing serious adverse effects, hematopoietic stem cell transplantation offers some hope [29]. However, it is very costly, and suitable donors are limited. Gene therapy and gene editing approaches [8], including CRISPR/Cas9 [30], which are being investigated for their use in treating genetic diseases, hold a great deal of promise for the future, if pursued with vigor, for the benefit and relief of these long-suffering victims of one of the most painful, debilitating, and deadly diseases in the history of medicine [31]. Note the 2017 news story from *Kaiser Health News*: "To sickle cell patients and their families—most of whom are African American—efforts to fight the disease appear slow, underfunded, ineffective or too limited in scope, perpetuating disparities that have existed for more than a century" [32]. But there is some good news on the horizon. As of late 2019, research on gene editing therapy for SCD has been advancing more rapidly, according to the Director of the NIH, Francis Collins [33] (Fig. 1.11). Do we dare dream of a cure?

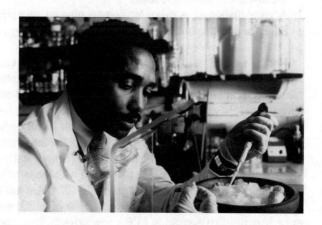

Fig. 1.11 Researcher at the National Heart, Lung, and Blood Institute engaged in the study of sickle cell anemia, 1987. (Courtesy NIH, National Library of Medicine)

Hypertension

Often called *high blood pressure*, this disease is a worldwide scourge that is particularly deadly for blacks, especially in the United States, where the economic cost of hypertensive disease was $76.6 billion in 2010 [34] and has continued to increase over the years. In 2010, hypertension was found to be the world-leading cause of death and disability-adjusted life-years (DALYs) and also was determined to be a larger contributor to cardiovascular events in women and African Americans than in whites. Over the past several years, several studies and clinical trials have been carried out in an attempt to establish a more evidence-based and precise framework on which to determine who should be labeled as hypertensive and how such individuals should be treated. The newly released 2017 *Guideline for the Prevention, Detection, Evaluation, and Management of High Blood Pressure in Adults: A Report of the American College of Cardiology/American Heart Association Task Force on Clinical Practice Guidelines* [34] is an update of the National Heart, Lung, and Blood Institute's *Seventh Report of the Joint National Committee on Prevention, Detection, Evaluation, and Treatment of High Blood Pressure* (JNC 7] published in 2004. The new report indicates that approximately 46% of the American population meet the criteria for hypertension, compared to 32% under previous guidelines, and that black patients require different treatment considerations than whites. According to Dr. Wilbert S. Aronow, a member of the 21-person committee that composed the new guidelines, "black patients have a higher prevalence of hypertension and adverse clinical outcomes than whites. Genetics and socioeconomic factors contribute to this. Blacks are also more salt-sensitive than whites" [35]. According to the new guidelines, hypertensive black adults who are at particular risk of the effects of the disease, such as those with co-morbidities such as diabetes, heart failure (HF), or kidney failure, should receive treatment with the following:

1. A thiazide diuretic (preferably chlorthalidone) or a calcium channel blocker as the first antihypertensive drug.
2. A combination of a thiazide diuretic plus an angiotensin-converting enzyme inhibitor or angiotensin receptor blocker, if three drugs are needed.

Not all patients will require drug treatment. Many can be managed with lifestyle changes such as dietary adjustments and increased physical activity. Treatment recommendations are different for white and other non-black patients with hypertension, and they vary according to age of the patient, i.e., whether the patient is younger or older than 60 years [36]. A complete list of updated criteria can be found in the published *2017 Guidelines* [28]. Using the new definition of hypertension as a level of blood pressure exceeding 130/80 (simply stated, 130 systolic is the new high), many more people will be diagnosed with the condition, which is a considerable change from the previous cut point of 140/90 that has been utilized since 1993. As an example, 59% of black men and 56% of black women are now estimated to be hypertensive according to the new criteria, compared to 47% of white men and 41% of white women in the United States. According to the new categories of

Table 1.1 Categories of blood pressure (BP) in adults [34]

BP category	Systolic BP (mmHg)		Diastolic BP (mmHg)
Normal	<120	and	<80
Elevated	120–129	and	<80
Hypertension			
Stage 1	130–139	or	80–89
Stage 2	≥140	or	≥90

Individuals with systolic BP and diastolic BP in two categories should be designated to the higher BP category
BP is based on ≥ two careful readings obtained on ≥ occasions

blood pressure in adults (Table 1.1), there are now three basic categories: normal, elevated BP, and hypertension, stage 1 and stage 2. Previous designations such as pre-hypertension and malignant hypertension have been eliminated [34].

The new hypertension guideline is associated with the use of the ACC/AHA Risk Calculator (http://www.cvriskcalculator.com/). It is important to determine risk in the case of minorities, especially African Americans. For instance, a 45-year-old who is free of hypertension has a 40-year risk of 93% if black, 92% if Hispanic, 86% if white, and 84% if Chinese American. The Risk Calculator can help to determine specific risk based in part on race, which was not a part of previous guidelines. However, Steve Nissen of the Cleveland Clinic cautions that care should be exercised in applying the ACC/AHA Risk Calculator that was devised for assessing risk in patients with elevated lipids to the hypertensive population, in as much as there has been no experience in utilizing this metric in minority populations [37].

Hypertension is more prevalent in African Americans than in other races and ethnic groups in the United States (Fig. 1.12) [38]. The disease tends to manifest different characteristics when it occurs in blacks. For instance, it is well known that the onset of hypertension may be at a young age and is often at a more advanced stage by the time of diagnosis. In addition, hypertension progresses to target organ damage much more rapidly in blacks than in whites and other races and ethnicities, is more difficult to control, and often leads to death at an early age [39, 40]. The mortality rate from hypertension is much higher in blacks than in whites. For these reasons, it is sensible to regard hypertension in blacks as a disease with multiple healthcare disparities. It must be approached in a different fashion concerning diagnosis, prevention, treatment, and management than in other racial and ethnic groups in order to optimize outcomes of appropriate therapeutic interventions [41].

Hypertension is a major risk factor for stroke, heart attack, renal failure, HF, and blindness, and this is especially true in blacks [42]. Efforts to reduce morbidity and mortality from these diseases must be linked to prevention and control of hypertension. There is a complex interrelationship of multiple factors involved in attempting to prevent and control the disease in the individual patient [43]. As elucidated by Bronfenbrenner in his ecological model (Fig. 1.13) [43, 44], the interplay of all of the factors displayed is important in the effort to reduce healthcare disparities that impact the patient. These are barriers that include the national health policy environment, which is undergoing drastic change at the present time as the nation undertakes a transition from Obamacare to another form of healthcare delivery, the

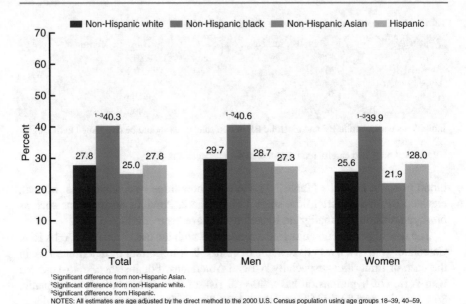

¹Significant difference from non-Hispanic Asian.
²Significant difference from non-Hispanic white.
³Significant difference from Hispanic.
NOTES: All estimates are age adjusted by the direct method to the 2000 U.S. Census population using age groups 18–39, 40–59, and 60 and over. Access data table for Figure 2 at: https://www.cdc.gov/nchs/data/databriefs/db289_table.pdf#2.
SOURCE: NCHS, National Health and Nutrition Examination Survey, 2015–2016.

Fig. 1.12 Age-adjusted prevalence of hypertension among adults aged 18 and over, by sex and race and Hispanic origin, United States, 2015–2016 (From Fryar et al. [38])

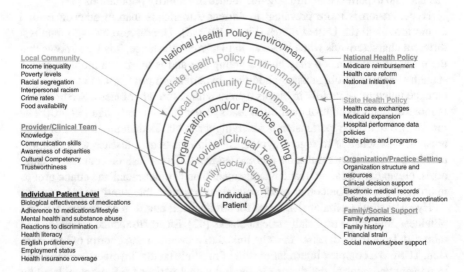

Fig. 1.13 Multilevel influences on disparities in hypertension prevention and control. (© American Journal of Hypertension, Ltd. 2014) (From Mueller et al. [43] with permission from Oxford University Press)

state health policy environment, the local community environment, the organization and/or practice setting, the provider/clinical team, and family/social support.

As was noted above, one of the principal problems in managing hypertension in blacks is *control*. Many epidemiological studies over the past several decades, including the National Health and Nutrition Examination Surveys (NHANES), have demonstrated the persistent difficulty with this critical aspect of hypertension management [38]. Although there has been some overall improvement in control of high blood pressure over the years, the goal of Healthy People 2020 of 61.2% control by 2020 was not met in the NHANES report of 2015–2016 (controlled hypertension was previously defined as a systolic pressure of less than 140 mmHg and a diastolic pressure of less than 90 mmHg among those with hypertension) [45], but as was discussed above, these cut points are changing with the appearance of the 2017 ACC/AHA Guideline).

A major factor in achieving hypertension control is *compliance* with taking medication. Adherence to medication decreases precipitously from the writing of a prescription to the taking of the medication and through the refilling of the prescription. Only 51% of patients being treated for hypertension in the United States follow the advice of healthcare professionals for long-term medical therapy. Lack of adherence can have deadly consequences, since nonadherence to medications for cardioprotection can increase a patient's risk of death from 50% to 80% [46].

Ferdinand et al. have indicated the importance of recognizing socioeconomic and cultural factors in attempting to increase compliance and to improve control hypertension in blacks [47]. They recommend eight different approaches to impacting this situation:

1. Patient engagement.
2. Consumer-directed healthcare.
3. Patient portals.
4. Smartphone apps.
5. Digital pillboxes and pill bottles.
6. Pharmacist-led engagement.
7. Cardiac rehabilitation.
8. Cognitive-based behavior.

Similarly, Mills et al. recommend a multilevel, multicomponent approach to control blood pressure in hypertensives. A meta-analysis research study showed that multilevel, multicomponent strategies, followed by patient-level strategies, are the most effective for controlling hypertension and should be used to effect better control [48].

If these and other measures are incorporated into a team approach to the hypertensive patient and if the one-size-fits-all concept is exchanged for a personalized approach that focuses on the unique characteristics of each patient, control of hypertension should improve. This change in the management of hypertensive black patients should be particularly beneficial to their health.

Innovative programs to increase awareness of hypertension include a model of hypertension care for black men that was recently reported by Ronald G. Victor, hypertension expert at the Cedars Sinai Medical Center in Los Angeles. (Sadly, Dr. Victor passed away on September 10, 2018, from pancreatic cancer.) As described in the *New England Journal of Medicine* [49], the "barbershop study" involved barbershops where black men go for haircuts; barbers were recruited, educated about high blood pressure and its dangers for the African American population, and were then asked to communicate this information to their clients, who were invited to enroll in this unique barbershop research program. Specifically, a cohort of 319 black male patrons with a systolic blood pressure of 140 mm Hg from 52 black-owned barbershops were enrolled in a cluster-randomized trial with two arms: one in which barbershops were assigned to a pharmacist-led intervention, in which barbers held meetings in barbershops with specialty-trained pharmacists who prescribed antihypertensive drug therapy to hypertensive clients in collaboration with the patients' physicians, and the other that was an active control approach in which lifestyle modifications and physicians' appointments were encouraged by the barbers. The primary outcome of the study of interventions in black men with uncontrolled hypertension was a reduction of systolic blood pressure at 6 months. This unconventional study of health promotion by barbers working with black barbershop patrons resulted in greater reduction of blood pressure when it was coupled with management of medication by specialty-trained pharmacists. The mean systolic blood pressure (MSP) at baseline was 152.8 mm Hg in the intervention group and 154.6 in the control group. At 6 months, the MSP in the intervention group was reduced 21.6 mm Hg more than in the control group. As a secondary blood pressure outcome, the mean diastolic pressure (MDP) was also reduced more in the intervention than in the control group, 14.9 mm Hg greater. There was a 95% retention rate in the intervention cohort.

This study represents an example of how preventive measures applied to a population at great risk of the ravages of hypertension can lead to greater control and may lead to saving lives. More than 200,000 deaths occur annually from preventable cardiovascular disease including hypertension. Since the risk of avoidable deaths from CVD is 80% higher in black men than in white males or black women [50], a particular emphasis should be placed on creating programs to control high blood pressure in black males. This investigation was very successful in achieving the primary outcome and gives promise of similar control of hypertension in blacks that should have a profound ripple effect across the cardiovascular disease spectrum.

Heart Failure

Background, Natural History, Epidemiology, and Pathophysiology

Sometimes called *congestive heart failure*, HF disproportionately affects African Americans much more than other subpopulations in the United States. That fact in and of itself identifies it as a healthcare disparity. The overall prevalence of the disease is 6.6 million people or almost 3% of the adult population. It is on the rise despite efforts to control it, and it is estimated that the prevalence will increase 25% by 2030 [51]. Blacks are especially impacted. The annual incidence of the disease in whites is about 6 per 1000 person-years compared to 9.1 per 1000 person-years in African Americans. The risk of death in blacks hospitalized for HF is 45% higher than for whites [52]. HF also occurs earlier in blacks than in whites; it occurs 20 times more frequently in blacks prior to age 50 than it does in whites, according to Bibbins-Domingo et al. [53].

The principal risk factor that predisposes blacks to HF is hypertension, which, as indicated above, predominates in African Americans as compared to Caucasians. Since hypertension is controllable, this means that the disparity that exists for HF in blacks can be reduced by controlling that condition. It must be understood that nothing is more important in preventing the onset and ravages of HF in blacks than controlling hypertension. From a pathophysiological viewpoint, hypertension leads to nonischemic cardiomyopathy as a prelude to HF in blacks, whereas whites develop ischemic cardiomyopathy as a result of coronary heart disease more commonly as the basis for their HF [54, 55]. Blacks also tend to develop HF with reduced ejection fraction (HFreF) more commonly than HF with preserved ejection fraction (HFpeF) [56].

Although hypertension predominates as the main precursor of HF in blacks, there are other factors that interdigitate in the mosaic that represents the disease. Included are obesity, chronic kidney disease, and diabetes, all of which are more common in blacks than in whites. Underlying all of these conditions is impaired endothelial dysfunction, which renders the arterial system in blacks less flexible than in whites. The relatively lower amount of elasticity in the arterial bed of blacks and the relative lack of responsiveness to vasodilators and nitric oxide as well as an increased responsiveness to vasoconstrictor agents have been documented [57, 58]. It is speculated that these pathophysiological abnormalities are the main causes of the greater propensity of blacks for HF.

Amyloidosis of the heart is another disease that tends to occur more commonly in blacks and is increasingly found as the cause of HF in this population [59, 60]. Transthyretin (TTR) is a 127-amino acid protein formed primarily in the liver, which circulates as a homo-tetramer due to genetic mutation, aging, or other causes; the tetramers may dissociate into monomers, which then become misfolded and become amyloid fibrils that may be deposited in several organs, including the heart. There are two types of amyloid that may infiltrate the heart: immunoglobulin light chain, called AL or primary systemic amyloid, and TTR amyloid. The latter, in turn, is comprised of two forms: familial or hereditary (hATTR) and wild-type (wtATTR or SSA, senile systemic amyloidosis which is sporadic in nature) [61]. In patients over the age of 60 years, hATTR occurs four times more frequently in African Americans than in Caucasians in its hereditary or familial form [62]. It is an infiltrative disorder that is progressive, often being misdiagnosed as hypertensive or hypertrophic cardiomyopathy. Its presence may be revealed by genetic testing, which can uncover the mutated TTR. Hereditary amyloidosis has been identified as occurring disproportionately in older black patients; it is transmitted in an autosomal dominant fashion leading to mutation of the TTR genome (ATTRmt). This is a point mutation that results in the substitution of isoleucine for valine at position 122 (Val 122lle) and leads to amyloid deposition that is predominately isolated to the heart. Investigation of living patients indicates that the mutation is highly prevalent in blacks, with an estimated 4% of the African American population being affected, which means that there may be more than 1.5 million blacks at risk of having this disease. This genetic mutation is virtually undetectable in the white population. A separate autopsy study showed that all black patients with the Val 122lle mutation had evidence of cardiac amyloid deposition (100% penetrance) [62].

It is important to recognize that the carrier or heterozygous state of this disease is associated with increased incidence of HF. Improved diagnostic techniques and effective therapies are being developed [62]. The electrocardiogram may demonstrate a classic pattern often seen in cardiac amyloidosis, which features low QRS voltage and a "pseudo-infarct" pattern with Q-wave and T-wave pattern suggestive of myocardial infarction. Cardiac arrhythmias, especially atrial fibrillation, may be seen. The echocardiogram may show progressive biventricular wall and atrial septal thickening, with loss of compliance and diastolic dysfunction. The myocardium has a "speckled" appearance, and signs of elevated filling pressures such as pleural and pericardial effusions may be seen on echo. In addition to genetic testing to detect gene mutations, imaging methods, including the use of the radioactive tracer technetium 99m pyrophosphate scan (PYP), cardiac magnetic resonance (CMR), and longitudinal strain measurement by tissue Doppler, may be helpful in diagnosing amyloid cardiomyopathy. Some red flag signs and symptoms include bilateral carpal tunnel syndrome; lumbar spinal stenosis; polyneuropathy symptoms such as burning, numbness, and tingling of the hands and feet; dizziness; ataxia; and orthostasis. Early diagnosis is important in order to give patients the benefit of earlier treatment, especially since the median survival time from diagnosis to death is 4.7 years. The Transthyretin Amyloidosis Cardiac Study (TRACS) found that survival after diagnosis was higher for SSA than for V121I patients (46 vs. 26 months, respectively) [63]. Treatment options are increasing for TTR cardiac amyloidosis. Recently, the FDA approved the use of tafamidis meglumine (Vyndaqel®) [64] for the disease. This drug binds to TTR, preventing dissociation of tetramers. It stabilizes myocardial amyloid infiltration, inhibits misfolding, and causes regression of wall thickness. Results of the ATTR-ACT Study of tafamidis showed a very significant decrease in mortality and hospitalizations [65]. Several other drugs are in the pipeline to treat this disease.

Preventing and Treating Heart Failure

Preventing HF is principally a matter of identifying modifiable risk factors and attempting to change them to benefit the patient. Examples include hypertension, which is the greatest risk factor in blacks, as described above. Other modifiable risk factors are obesity, diabetes, smoking, dyslipidemia, alcoholism, physical inactivity, valvular heart disease, and improper diet such as eating foods with a high salt content.

Treatment of HF has seen a long and convoluted history that is still developing. One of the earliest drugs used in this disease is digitalis, which was a mainstay several years ago but has recently fallen into disfavor, except in special circumstances, because of relative lack of effectiveness in decreasing overall mortality, although it was found to reduce hospitalizations for worsening HF. It has also been documented to be even less effective in black patients in lowering mortality, as was seen in the Digitalis Investigation Group study, a randomized clinical trial of the drug, in which 14% of the study participants were black [66].

Over the course of the years, several paradigms of HF treatment have evolved, none of which has substantially reduced the ravages of this deadly disease. It still exacts a mortality toll amounting to 50% of its victims dying within 5 years of diagnosis. As was stated, black patients have the shortest survival when they are stricken with HF and the least benefit from the numerous medications and devices that are used [67].

A new drug was approved by the FDA in 2015 which has given great hope in the treatment of HF with reduced ejection fraction. Called Entresto (Novartis, East Hanover NJ, USA), it is a combination of two medications: *valsartan*, an angiotensin II receptor blocker (ARB), and the endopeptidase *sacubitril*, a neprilysin (NEP) inhibitor that metabolizes various vasoactive peptides. In the PARADIGM-HF study in which more than 8000 patients with New York Heart Association (NYHA) classes II–IV HF were given either Entresto or enalapril (the established treatment), there was a dramatic 20% reduction of the risk of death, which was the primary endpoint; and there was also a corresponding 21% decrease in HF hospitalizations, as well as a 16% decrease in all-cause mortality. In fact, these results were so impressive that the PARADIGM-HF trial was stopped after 27 months for ethical reasons [68]. Special consideration of the use of this very effective drug in black patients is necessary because only 5% of the total patients recruited were African American. It is well known that blacks have a propensity to developing angioedema when treated with angiotensin-converting enzyme (ACE) inhibitors [69] and also with ARBs such as valsartan; there was some concern that this might become a problem in the study if a larger number of blacks were involved as subjects. Therefore, questions have arisen about whether Entresto has been sufficiently vetted as a drug that can safely be administered to black patients. The evidence base for such a determination is weak. This is not to say that Entresto should not be used to treat HF in black patients; the recommendation is to use it in this population with an abundance of caution.

There are certain standards of care for HF that apply to most patients, including blacks. The standard drugs that are used include beta-blockers, ACE inhibitors, ARBs, and aldosterone antagonists. There may be differences in drug effectiveness between blacks and whites; one meta-analysis by Shekelle et al. showed less effectiveness of ACEs and beta-blockers in the treatment of left ventricular systolic dysfunction in black patients [70]. There are also some differential concerns regarding adverse effects such as angioedema which is 3–4% higher in blacks treated with ACEs [71, 72].

Regarding survival of black compared to white patients hospitalized for HF, Deswal et al. [73] found better survival of black patients after hospitalization, although she could not attribute this to differences in healthcare utilization. It should be emphasized that this was a large retrospective study of hospitalized patients; the results showing better survival of blacks is in contradistinction to studies of patients outside of the hospital such as in communities, which tend to show lesser survival in blacks with HF [74].

Perhaps the biggest issue regarding the treatment of HF in blacks concerns the use of BiDil (Arbor Pharmaceuticals, Atlanta GA, USA), a fixed-dose combination of two vasodilators, hydralazine hydrochloride and isosorbide dinitrate, which was approved by the FDA in 2005 for the treatment of black patients with New York Heart Association class II or class IV HF. The African American Heart Failure Trial (A-HEFT), organized by the Association of Black Cardiologists and led by Anne L. Taylor, University of Minnesota, was a blockbuster study that was characterized by a 43% reduction in all-cause mortality, a 39% decrease in the risk of a first hospitalization for HF, and an improvement in functional status that was statistically significant as measured by the self-administer *Minnesota Living with Heart Failure* questionnaire [75]. Patients who qualified for this unique study, all of whom were self-identified African Americans, had not been hospitalized for HF before and were receiving background therapy, including neurohormonal blockers and other medications.

After BiDil entered the marketplace, it languished and was not used by physicians treating black HF patients to the extent that was expected of a drug with such evidence-based documentation of its effectiveness for blacks. This was despite the fact that in 2005, the American College of Cardiology and the American Heart Association stated in their guideline update for the diagnosis and management of chronic HF in the adult, that "the addition of isosorbide dinitrate and hydralazine to a standard medical regimen for HF, including [angiotensin-converting enzyme inhibitors] and beta-blockers, is reasonable and can be effective in blacks with [New York Heart Association] functional class II or IV HF" [76]. In addition, in 2006, the Heart Failure Society of America updated its comprehensive HF practice guideline, stating that "A strong recommendation now exists for the addition of the fixed combination of Isosorbide dinitrate and hydralazine to the standard medical regimen for African Americans with HF" [77]. Although there have been more recent recommendations and guidelines from authoritative cardiological societies for use of BiDil in blacks with HF, the usage rate continues to lag behind. Fonarow et al. estimated that 27% of blacks with HF in the United States were eligible to receive BiDil in 2011, but only a small percentage actually were treated with it. They suggested that if the medication were dispensed appropriately, there could be a large implementation benefit for blacks with HF in terms of a reduction in mortality [78]. It should be apparent that African Americans with HF are not receiving the standard of care and are dying because of a healthcare disparity that could be reduced or eliminated if a quality improvement initiative were put in place.

Opioid Addiction

The United States is currently struggling with a crisis of addiction to opioid drugs. The rate of opioid abuse has increased 500% since 1999 and therefore must be considered to be of epidemic proportions (Figs. 1.14 and 1.15).

It must be made clear that that addiction to opioid drugs is a major threat to the very survival of the African American community, if not to our entire society. This is not hyperbole. The history of opioid addiction in the general population will be reviewed first.

Addiction to opioid drugs is not new in America, but it has proliferated alarmingly in recent years and is now considered to be an epidemic. There were 42,249 opioid-overdose deaths in the United States in 2016, which is a 28% increase in 1 year. According to the National Center for Health Statistics, the dramatic surge

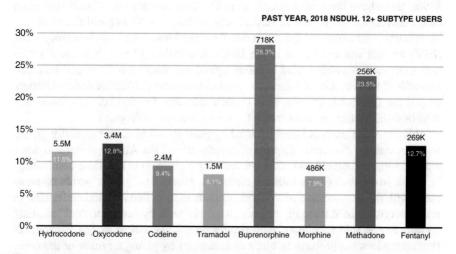

Fig. 1.14 Misuse of prescription opioid subtypes. US Department of Health. Human Services. Substance Abuse and Mental Health Services Administration. 2018 National Survey on Drug Use and Health. http://www.samhsa.gov/data/data-we-collect/nsduh-national-survey-drug-use-and-health. Accessed 27 Dec 2019

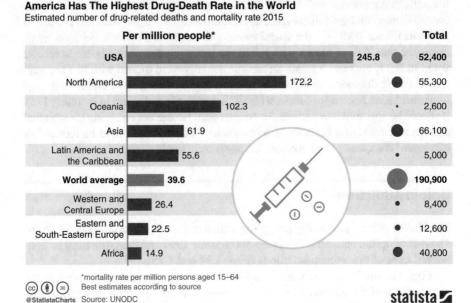

America Has The Highest Drug-Death Rate in the World
Estimated number of drug-related deaths and mortality rate 2015

Per million people*		Total
USA	245.8	52,400
North America	172.2	55,300
Oceania	102.3	2,600
Asia	61.9	66,100
Latin America and the Caribbean	55.6	5,000
World average	**39.6**	**190,900**
Western and Central Europe	26.4	8,400
Eastern and South-Eastern Europe	22.5	12,600
Africa	14.9	40,800

*mortality rate per million persons aged 15–64
Best estimates according to source
@StatistaCharts Source: UNODC

statista

Fig. 1.15 Statista Charts. Drug-related deaths and mortality rate worldwide. Data source: United Nations Office of Drugs and Crime. https://www.statista.com/chart/9973/drug-related-deaths-and-mortality-rate-worldwide/. Statista Chart CC BY-SA 3.0. Accessed 27 Dec 2019

in unintentional deaths, of which opioid-overdose deaths are part, has caused a 2-year decline in life expectancy for the first time since the 1960s [79]. Since the 1990s, there have been more deaths annually from overdose of opioids than from motor vehicle accidents, and 115 lives a day are lost to it. The opioid abuse mortality rate has even exceeded the death rate from the human immunodeficiency virus (HIV) when it was at its peak in the 1990s. It is estimated that there are 2.1 million Americans who have what is called opioid use disorder (OUD), and less than one-fifth of them receive medication-assisted treatment (MAT) for their addiction, despite the fact that it has proven to be very effective. Put another way, more than 80% of OUD victims go untreated [80]. This is a national disgrace.

This overdose crisis is largely caused by poor access to care, especially office-based treatment. The crisis disproportionately affects the African American community. Although opioid addiction was initially a problem in the white community, in recent years blacks have become victims in greater and greater numbers, especially with the proliferation of synthetic opioids such as fentanyl and carfentanil (a very powerful animal tranquilizer), which may be used by dealers to "cut" or dilute cocaine that is sold to addicts, with deadly results. An article in *The Washington Post* epitomizes the problem in black communities by giving a profile of the crisis in Cleveland, Ohio, in 2017. Of 399 fentanyl-related deaths in Cuyahoga County, 58 were black addicts. This was a marked increase from previous patterns and is believed to be due to the admixture of fentanyl and cocaine sold to black addicts in particular. This caused a doubling of African American-related fentanyl deaths in 1 year, between 2016 and 2017, and a 900% increase between 2014 and 2016 [81]. Additionally, in December 2017, *The New York Times*, citing data from the Centers for Disease Control and Prevention (CDC), reported that "Drug deaths in urban counties rose by 41% in 2016, far outpacing any other racial or ethnic group" [82]. This identifies opioid overdosing as a healthcare disparity that is very much in need of fixing.

Fortunately, Congress has recognized that there is a crisis of OUD and has taken steps to eliminate it [83]. In fiscal 2018, Congress appropriated an additional $500 million to the National Institutes of Health (NIH) budget to advance their plan called Helping to End Addiction Long-term (HEAL) [84]. This is described as an action-oriented research plan that is focused on improving treatment for opioid use and addiction and enhancing pain management strategies (Table 1.2). The initiative will start with the Healing Communities Study, a multisite program that will measure the effect of what is termed integrated implementation of a comprehensive set of evidence-based strategies of prevention, screening, detection, treatment, and retention in treatment. HEAL's complex plan also contains a new public-private

Table 1.2 National Institutes of Health Helping to End Addiction Long-Term (HEAL) initiative research plan: Deliverables and timeline [84]

In the short term (within 3–5 years), HEAL research investments are expected to deliver:
 Implementation strategies demonstrated to significantly increase initiation of medication-based treatment and retention in treatment beyond 6 months and to decrease rates of opioid addiction and overdose death
 Biological signatures to predict which patients are at risk for developing chronic pain, guiding precision medicine approaches to reduce patient transition to chronic pain and thereby reducing reliance on opioids
 A comprehensive dataset for the research community to reveal factors that predict transition or resilience to chronic pain
 Identification of novel targets associated with spinal and peripheral pain pathways
 A clinical trial network poised for the rapid testing of new pain therapies
 New evidence-based approaches to inform previous practice-based approaches and improve care for infants with neonatal opioid withdrawal syndrome
 Evidence for the nonpharmacological management of multiple acute and chronic pain conditions
In the longer term (over 5 years), HEAL will deliver:
 Pharmaceutical programs leading to 15 investigational new drug applications and investigational device exemptions, with the goal of 5 new drug applications or 510 K/premarket approvals for devices submitted to the US Food and Drug Administration for:
  Overdose reversal agents
  More flexible and new medications for the treatment of opioid use disorder
  New interventions against respiratory depression to stop overdose death
  Novel medications to treat withdrawal, craving, and relapse
  Increased options for small molecules, biologics, and neuromodulation devices for the treatment of pain without the use of opioids
  A pipeline of novel non-opioid therapies that can be further developed and tested for the treatment of acute and chronic pain
  Understanding of the lasting effects of early exposure to opioids on children and young adults

partnership working with patients in a "hub-and-spoke" arrangement of clinical trials. Hopefully, this innovative paradigm will provide the type of precision medicine needed to heal the nation by ridding it of the deadly scourge of OUD.

Another area of concern is the use of opioids for the treatment of chronic pain. Buprenorphine, a partial agonist-antagonist of the mu receptor in the brain, is a synthetic opioid that should be considered for pain management over more addictive drugs. Naltrexone, an antagonist, and methadone, an opioid agonist, are also useful in medically assisted treatment of OUD and have been shown to reduce the addictive consequences of OUD. However, they are underutilized. Proper use depends in part on removal of the stigma associated with treating addiction. Doing so has the potential of saving thousands of lives through overdose prevention, which must become a national priority.

A barrier to rescuing addicts from overdose deaths involves the criminal justice system; 14 states currently threaten criminal prosecution of physicians who distribute the overdose-reversal drug naloxone to individuals without a prescription, and 36 states make possession of this potentially life-saving drug without a prescription illegal. The United States can take a lesson from Canada, which has reduced the unsafe prescribing of opioids for pain relief by making naloxone and other drugs publicly available, and when indicated, free of charge [85]. Other innovative programs that have life-saving potential such as the provision of supervised injection sites for addicts are being considered in an effort to bring the deadly scourge of narcotics addiction and OUD under control. However, more physicians are needed to help control these problems; currently, only 4% of physicians eligible to treat opioid addiction have received the waiver required by the federal government to prescribe medication-assisted treatment.

Human Immunodeficiency Virus (HIV)/Acquired Immunodeficiency Syndrome (AIDS)

It is an oversimplification to state that HIV/AIDS disproportionately affects African Americans; in fact, this deadly disease has been extremely devastating to blacks. Consider the numbers and statistics [86]:

1. Although blacks comprise about 12% of the American population, they make up 44% of the HIV diagnoses.
2. In 2016, 17,528 blacks were diagnosed with HIV: 12,890 men and 4,560 women.
3. 47% of those diagnosed with AIDS in 2016 were black.
4. African Americans account for a higher percentage of newly diagnosed cases and of those living with HIV, which amounts to 1.2 million people. At the end of 2014, it is estimated that 471,500 African Americans were living with HIV, and 1 in 6 were unaware of this status.
5. Six out of 10 blacks diagnosed with HIV were gay or bisexual men.
6. In 2015, 3,379 blacks died from HIV disease, which accounted for 52% of deaths attributed to the disease.

History of HIV/AIDS in the United States

The origin of this disease is controversial. It may have originated in certain parts of Africa in the early part of the twentieth century. The earliest documented appearance in the United States was in 1971 in New York City; it then spread to other large cities including San Francisco and mainly infected intravenous drug abusers and gay men [87].

Diagnosis

It should be noted that HIV is diagnosed separately from AIDS. HIV is detected in bodily fluids such as serum, semen, vaginal fluid, urine, and saliva. Testing is performed to detect HIV antibodies to the HIV antigens. The ELISA (enzyme-linked immunosorbent assay) test, which is highly sensitive, is performed first, followed by the Western blot test and other laboratory analyses as necessary. The diagnosis of AIDS, which occurs at a later stage of HIV infection, is based on further laboratory testing (decreased CD4 count, under 200 cells) and/or the appearance of a number of clinical symptoms and signs (presence of cancers, i.e., Kaposi's sarcoma, lymphoma, anal cancer, or infections such as *Pneumocystis jirovecii (formerly carinii)* pneumonia [PCP], tuberculosis, body rash, etc.).

Pathophysiology and Epidemiology

AIDS is caused by the human immune deficiency virus, of which there are two strains, HIV-1, the more virulent type that is found in most cases, and HIV-2. The disease is now global in its distribution and is still considered to be an epidemic in the United States, where 1.2 million people are living with HIV. A disproportionate burden is carried by African Americans and by men who have sex with men [88].

Progress in Treatment and Management of HIV/AIDS

Treatment of this disease has been very successful since very potent antiretroviral therapy was developed in 1996. During this time interval, the strategy of *treatment as prevention* was initiated. The goal was to achieve complete viral suppression in at least 73% of HIV patients. This goal was based on the results of the international, groundbreaking HPTN 052 clinical trial (https://www.hptn.org/), which determined that sustaining viral suppression can eliminate heterosexual transmission. This gave researchers hope that viral suppression might end the HIV/AIDS epidemic. According to Anthony S. Fauci, MD, Director of the NIH National Institute of Allergy and Infectious Diseases, complete suppression of the viral load in HIV/AIDS patients has the prospect of eliminating the epidemic in the course of a generation.

However, there are problems with accomplishing this goal. Nance et al. [88] has called the main problem an implementation gap, i.e., there are healthcare disparities in suppressing viral load in all populations. Although there have been gains in viral load suppression since 1997, there is not an equal distribution across all groups. In particular, there is a persistence of detectable viral loads in blacks as opposed to other races and ethnicities. This is a gap that could have deadly consequences and should be investigated.

Another approach to the HIV/AIDS crisis is prevention. Pre-exposure prophylaxis (PrEP) is an innovative initiative that began about 6 years ago for the purpose of treating the HIV-negative partners of HIV-positive individuals with antiretroviral therapy in the hope of stemming the spread of the disease. The drug prophylaxis approach, which was premiered in Botswana [89], was approved for that purpose by the FDA in 2012 [90]. This preventive strategy, which utilizes oral tenofovir disoproxil fumarate, has proven safe and highly effective [91] and is felt to have the potential of stemming the HIV/AIDS epidemic. However, there is a disparity in its use in that some communities that need it the most are not fully accepting it. For example, although blacks constituted 45% of the new HIV infections in the United States in 2015, only 10% of the PrEP users between 2012 and 2015 were black, as compared to a 74% utilization rate among whites who represented 27% of new infections [92, 93].

A number of studies have shown that blacks, who are the group at highest risk, are the least likely to use this very powerful, safe, and effective tool for the prevention of HIV infection and to begin PrEP after initial engagement [94]. The putative reasons for this paradoxical phenomenon are numerous and include lack of awareness, fear, stigma, and lack of clinician recommendation. Interestingly, lack of insurance coverage does not seem to influence the decision to initiate PrEP. Referral source also matters; HIV rapid testing in health centers may have a low percentage of patients going on to initiate prophylaxis [94]. Lack of utilization of this resource must be reversed in order to save lives and to allow us to progress toward the total elimination of HIV/AIDS. Increased awareness of its availability, safety, and ease of administration must become a goal of every public health clinic and professional.

Australia is providing the best example in the world of the value of PrEP. They have made great inroads into the incidence of new cases of HIV/AIDS; in 2018 there were only 835 diagnoses compared to their peak year of 1987, when 2412 cases were diagnosed, according to a recent article in *The New York Times*, and they have realistic expectations of eliminating the disease altogether by 2030 [95]. They provide emtricitabine-tenofovir (Truvada®, Gilead, Foster City, CA, USA) free or at very low cost to citizens at risk and have observed an almost 100% rate of effectiveness in those who take it. As a result of their aggressive approach, it is estimated that only 0.1% of the population has the virus, compared to the United States, where the rate is four times higher. There is evidence that the same benefit could occur in the United States; some cities such as San Francisco and New York are seeing declines in prevalence rates, ostensibly because they are providing the drug free or subsidized. The hope is that more cities will follow Australia's example. Another combination of the same drugs with different concentrations of the components, Descovy®, is also used for PrEP.

Conclusion

This chapter has examined five critical healthcare problems that have an overarching impact on the very survival of blacks in the United States. The author began with these particular diseases in order to provide a sense of how serious healthcare delivery is and how it can vary according to race and ethnicity. Imagine these conditions diffused among 25 million African Americans, who receive substandard treatment and almost no preventive care for them. Imagine what impact having one of these conditions has on individuals and their families. And imagine the possibilities of improved health status and survival if healthcare disparities were eliminated. Eradicating barriers to access and developing a value-based system will allow us to realize the promise of true equity in healthcare delivery across all races and ethnicities. It is within our sights.

References

1. Williams RA, editor. Textbook of black-related diseases. New York: McGraw-Hill; 1975.
2. Herrick JB. Peculiar elongated and sickle-shaped red blood corpuscles in a case of severe anemia. Arch Intern Med. 1910;6(5):517–21.
3. Pauling L, Itano HA, Singer SJ, Wells IC. Sickle cell anemia, a molecular disease. Science. 1949;110(2865):543–8.
4. Al-Salem A. Genetics and pathophysiology of sickle cell anemia. In: Medical and surgical complications of sickle cell anemia. Cham, Switzerland: Springer International; 2016.
5. Bunn HF. Pathogenesis and treatment of sickle cell disease. N Engl J Med. 1997;337(11):762–9.
6. Ballas SK, Gupta K, Adams-Graves P. Sickle cell pain: a critical reappraisal. Blood. 2012;120(18):3647–56.
7. Kato GJ, Piel FB, Reid CD, Gaston MH, Ohene-Frempong K, Krishnamurti L, et al. Sickle cell disease. Nat Rev Dis Primers. 2018;4:18010. https://doi.org/10.1038/nrdp.2018.10. Review
8. Rees DC, Williams TN, Gladwin MT. Sickle cell disease. Lancet. 2010;376(9757):2018–31.
9. Piel FB, Steinberg MH, Rees DC. Sickle cell disease. N Engl J Med. 2017;376(16):1561–73.
10. Hassell KL. Population estimates of sickle cell disease in the U.S. Am J Prev Med. 2010;38(4 Suppl):S512–21.
11. Piel FB, Patil AP, Howes RE, Nyangiri OA, Gething PW, Dewi M, et al. Global epidemiology of sickle haemoglobin in neonates: a contemporary geostatistical model-based map and population estimates. Lancet. 2013;381(9861):142–51.
12. Centers of Disease Control and Prevention. Sickle cell trait fact sheet. http://www.cdc.gov/ncbddd/sicklecell/traits.html. Accessed 12 Sep 2019.
13. Lorey FW, Arnopp J, Cunningham GC. Distribution of hemoglobinopathy variants by ethnicity in a multiethnic state. Genet Epidemiol. 1996;13(5):501–12.
14. McCurdy PR. 32-DFP and 51-Cr for measurement of red cell life span in abnormal hemoglobin syndromes. Blood. 1969;33(2):214–24.
15. Tantawy AG. The scope of clinical morbidity in sickle cell trait. Egypt J Med Hum Genet. 2014;15(4):319–26.
16. Harris KM, Haas TS, Eichner RE, Maron BJ. Sickle cell trait associated with sudden death in competitive athletes. Am J Cardiol. 2012;110(8):1184–8.
17. Goldsmith JC, Bonham VL, Joiner CH, Kato GJ, Noonan AS, Steinberg MH. Framing the research agenda for sickle cell trait: building on the current understanding of clinical events and their potential implications. Am J Hematol. 2012;87(3):340–6.

18. Sullivan LW. The risks of sickle cell trait: caution and common sense. N Engl J Med. 1987;31(13):830–1.
19. Pauling LC. Reflections on the new biology. UCLA Law Rev. 1968;15:268–72.
20. Strouse JJ, Lobner K, Lanzkron S, Haywood C Jr. NIH and national foundation expenditures for sickle cell disease are associated with PUBMED publications and FDA approvals. Blood. 2013;122(21):739. http://www.bloodjournal.org/content/122/21/1739
21. Wong TE, Brandow AM, Lim W, Lortenberg R. Update on the use of hydroxyurea therapy in sickle cell disease. Blood. 2014;124(26):3850–7. quiz 4004
22. Gaston MH, Verter JI, Woods G, Pegelow C, Kelleher J, Presbury G, et al. Prophylaxis with oral penicillin in children with sickle cell anemia—a randomized trial. N Engl J Med. 1986;314(25):1593–9.
23. Figueiredo M. Endari reduces pain crises, hospitalizations in sickle cell patients, phase 3 trial shows. Sickle Cell Anemia News. 26 Jul 2018.
24. Niihara Y, Miller ST, Kanter J, Lanzkron S, Smith WR, Hsu LL, et al. A phase 3 trial of l-glutamine in sickle cell disease. N Engl J Med. 2018;379(3):226–35.
25. Ataga KI, Kutlar A, Kanter J, Liles D, Cancado R, Friedrisch J, et al. Crizanlizumab for the prevention of pain crises in sickle cell disease. N Engl J Med. 2017;376(5):429–39.
26. Global Blood Therapeutics. GBT announces U.S. Food and Drug Administration acceptance of new drug application and priority review for voxelotor for the treatment of sickle cell disease. https://ir.gbt.com/news-releases/news-release-details/gbt-announces-us-food-and-drug-administration-acceptance-new. Accessed 9 Sep 2019.
27. Vichinsky E, Hoppe CC, Ataga KI, Ware RE, Nduba V, El-Beshlawy A, HOPE Trial Investigators, et al. A phase 3 randomized trial of voxelotor in sickle cell disease. N Engl J Med. 2019;381(6):509–19.
28. Adams RJ, McKie VC, Hsu L, Files B, Vichinsky E, Pegelow C, et al. Prevention of a first stroke by transfusion in children with sickle cell anemia and abnormal results on transcranial Doppler ultrasonography. N Engl J Med. 1998;339(1):5–11.
29. Hsieh MM, Fitzhugh CD, Weitzel RP, Link ME, Coles WA, Zhao X, et al. Nonmyeloablative HLA-matched sibling allogeneic hematopoietic stem cell transplantation for severe sickle cell phenotype. JAMA. 2014;312(1):48–56.
30. Hoban MD, Orkin SH, Bauer DE. Genetic treatment of a molecular disorder: gene therapy approaches to sickle cell disease. Blood. 2016;127(7):839–48.
31. Zhang F, Wen Y, Guo X. CRISPR/Cas9 for genome editing: progress, implications, and challenges. Hum Mol Genet. 2014;23(R1):R40–6.
32. Gold J. Sickle cell patients, families and doctors face a "fight for everything." Kaiser Health News. 27 Dec 2017. https://khn.org/news/sickle-cell-patients-families-and-doctors-face-a-fight-for-everything/. Accessed 11 Sep 2019.
33. Lapook J. Could gene therapy cure sickle cell anemia? 60 Minutes. 29 Dec 2019. https://https://www.cbsnews.com/news/more-on-the-trial-aiming-to-cure-sickle-cell-60-minutes-2019-12-29/. Accessed 4 Jan 2020.
34. Whelton PK, Carey RM, Aronow WS, Casey DE Jr, Collins KJ, Dennison Himmelfarb C, et al. 2017 ACC/AHA/AAPA/ABC/ACPM/AGS/APhA/ASH/ASPC/NMA/PCNA guideline for the prevention, detection, evaluation, and management of high blood pressure in adults: executive summary: a report of the American College of Cardiology/American Heart Association Task Force on Clinical Practice Guidelines. Hypertension. 2018;71(6):1269–324. Erratum in Hypertension. 2018;71(6):e136–9
35. Aronow WS. Initiation of antihypertensive therapy. Presented at American Heart Association (AHA) Scientific Session 2017; 11–15 Nov 2017; Anaheim, CA. https://www.abstractsonline.com/pp8/#!/4412/presentation/55060.
36. Howard G, Lackland DT, Kleindorfer DO, Kissela BM, Moy CS, Judd SE, et al. Racial differences in the impact of elevated systolic blood pressure on stroke risk. JAMA Intern Med. 2013;173(1):46–51.
37. Fleming M. Steven Nissen, MD: risk calculation is a risky business. MD Magazine. 31 Nov 2018. https://www.mdmag.com/conference-coverage/aha-2018/steven-nissen-md-risk-calculation-is-a-risky-business. Accessed 12 Sep 2018.

38. Fryar CD, Ostchega Y, Hales CM, Zhang G, Kruszon-Moran D. Hypertension prevalence and control among adults: United States, 2015–2016. NCHS data brief, no 289. Hyattsville, MD: National Center for Health Statistics. 2017.
39. Gibbs CR, Beevers DG, Lip GY. The management of hypertensive disease in black patients. QJM. 1999;92(4):187–92. Review
40. Lloyd-Jones D, Adams RJ, Brown TM, Carnethon M, Dai S, De Simone G, American Heart Association Statistics Committee and Stroke Statistics Subcommittee, et al. Heart disease and stroke statistics: 2010 update: a report from the American Heart Association. Circulation. 2010;121(7):e46–e215.
41. Wright JT Jr, Agadoa LY, Appel L, Cushman WC, Taylor AL, Obegdegbe GG, et al. New recommendations for treating hypertension in black patients: evidence and/or consensus? Hypertension. 2010;56(5):801–3.
42. Moulton SA. Hypertension in African Americans and its related chronic diseases. J Cult Divers. 2009;16(4):165–70.
43. Mueller M, Purnell TS, Mensah GA, Cooper LA. Reducing racial and ethnic disparities in hypertension prevention and control: what will it take to translate research into practice and policy? Am J Hypertens. 2015;28(6):699–716.
44. Bronfenbrenner U. Ecological models of human development. In: International encyclopedia of education, vol. Vol 3. 2nd ed. Oxford UK: Elsevier; 1994.
45. U.S. Department of Health and Human Services, Office of Disease Prevention and Health Promotion. Healthy People 2020. https://www.healthypeople.gov/. Accessed 12 Sep 2019.
46. Ho PM, Bryson CL, Rumsfeld JS. Medication adherence: its importance in cardiovascular outcomes. Circulation. 2009;119(23):3028–35.
47. Ferdinand KC, Yadav K, Nasser SA, Clayton-Jeter HD, Lewin J, Cryer DR, Senatore FF. Disparities in hypertension and cardiovascular disease in blacks: the critical role of medication adherence. J Clin Hypertens (Greenwich). 2017;19(10):1015–24.
48. Mills KT, Obst KM, Shen W, Molina S, Zhang HJ, He H, et al. Comparative effectiveness of implementation strategies for blood pressure control in hypertensive patients: a systematic review and meta-analysis. Ann Intern Med. 2018;168(2):110–20.
49. Victor RG, Lynch K, Li N, Blyler C, Muhammad E, Handler J, et al. A cluster-randomized trial of blood pressure reduction in black barbershops. N Engl J Med. 2018;378(14):1291–301.
50. Centers for Disease Control and Prevention. Vital signs: avoidable deaths from heart disease, stroke, and hypertensive disease – United States, 2001–2010. MMWR Morb Mortal Wkly Rep. 2013;62(35):721–7.
51. Go AS, Mozaffarian D, Roger VL, Benjamin EJ, Berry JD, Borden WB, American Heart Association Statistics Committee and Stroke Statistics Subcommittee, et al. American Heart Association Heart disease and stroke statistics—2013 update: a report from the American Heart Association. Circulation. 2013;127(1):e6–e245. Erratum in: Circulation. 2013;127(1). https://doi.org/10.1161/CIR.0b013e31828124ad. Circulation. 2013;127(23):e841
52. Bardy GH, Lee KL, Mark DB, Poole JE, Packer DL, Boineau R, Sudden Cardiac Death in Heart Failure Trial (SCD-HeFT) Investigators, et al. Amiodarone or an implantable cardioverter-defibrillator for congestive heart failure. N Engl J Med. 2005;352(3):225–37.
53. Bibbins-Domingo K, Pletcher MJ, Lin F, Vittinghoff E, Gardin JM, Arynchyn A, et al. Racial differences in incident heart failure among young adults. N Engl J Med. 2009;360(12):1179–90.
54. Bahrami H, Kronmal R, Bluemke DA, Olson J, Shea S, Liu K, et al. Differences in the incidence of congestive heart failure by ethnicity: the multi-ethnic study of atherosclerosis. Arch Intern Med. 2008;168(19):2138–45.
55. Loehr LR, Rosamond WD, Chang PP, Folsom AR, Chambless LE. Heart failure incidence and survival (from the Atherosclerosis Risk in Communities study). Am J Cardiol. 2008;101(7):1016–122.
56. Duprez DA, Jacobs DR Jr, Lutsey PL, Herrington D, Prime D, Ouyang P, et al. Race/ethnic and sex differences in large and small artery elasticity—results of the multi-ethnic study of atherosclerosis (MESA). Ethn Dis. 2009;19(1):243–50.
57. Kalinowski L, Dobrucki IT, Malinski T. Race-specific differences in endothelial function: predisposition of African Americans to vascular diseases. Circulation. 2004;109(21):2511–7.

58. Mulukutla SR, Venkitachalam L, Bambs C, Kip KE, Aiyer A, Marroquin OC, Reis SE. Black race is associated with digital artery endothelial dysfunction: results from the Heart SCORE study. Eur Heart J. 2010;31(22):2808–15.
59. Jacobson DR, Pastore RD, Yaghoubian R, Kane I, Gallo G, Buck FS, Buxbaum JN. Variant-sequence transthyretin (isoleucine 122) in late-onset cardiac amyloidosis in black Americans. N Engl J Med. 1997;336(7):466–73.
60. Buxbaum J, Alexander A, Koziol J, Tagoe C, Fox E, Kitzman D. Significance of the amy-loidogenic transthyretin val 122 lle allele in African Americans in the Atherosclerotic Risk in Communities (ARIC) and Cardiovascular Health (CHS) studies. Am Heart J. 2010;159(5):864–70.
61. Ruberg FL, Berk JL. Transthyretin(TTR) cardiac amyloidosis. Circulation. 2012;126(10):1286–300.
62. Shah KB, Mankad AK, Castano A, Akinboboye OO, Duncan PB, Fergus IV, Maurer MS. Transthyretin cardiac amyloidosis in black Americans. Circ Heart Fail. 2016;9(6):e00258.
63. Ruberg FL, Maurer M, Judge D, Zeldenrust S, Skinner M, Kim AY, et al. Prospective evalu-ation of the morbidity and mortality of wild-type and V122I mutant transthyretin amy-loid cardiomyopathy: the Transthyretin Amyloidosis Cardiac Study (TRACS). Am Heart J. 2012;64(2):222–8.
64. Maurer MS, Grogan DR, Judge DP. Tafamidis in transthyretin amyloid cardiomyopathy: effects on transthyretin stabilization and clinical outcomes. Circ Heart Fail. 2015;8(3):9629–34.
65. Maurer MS, Schwartz JH, Gundapaneni B, Elliott PM, Merlini G, Waddington-Cruz M, et al. Tafamidis treatment for patients with transthyretin amyloid cardiomyopathy. N Engl J Med. 2018;379(11):1007–16.
66. Digitalis Investigation Group. The effect of digoxin on mortality and morbidity in patients with heart failure. N Engl J Med. 1997;336(8):525–33.
67. Franciosa JA, Ferdinand KC, Yancy CW, Consensus Statement on Heart Failure in African Americans Writing Group. Treatment of heart failure in African Americans: a consensus state-ment. Congest Heart Fail. 2010;16(1):27–38.
68. Kaplinsky E. Sacubatril/valsartan in heart failure: latest evidence and place in therapy. Ther Adv Chronic Dis. 2016;7(6):278–90.
69. Brown N, Ray W, Snowden M, Griffin M. Black Americans have an increased rate of angiotensin converting enzyme inhibitor-associated angioedema. Clin Pharmacol Ther. 1996;60(1):8–13.
70. Shekelle PG, Rich MW, Morton SC, Atkinson CS, Tu W, Maglione M, et al. Efficacy of angio-tensin converting enzyme inhibitors and beta-blockers in the management of left ventricular systolic dysfunction according to race, gender, and diabetic status: a meta-analysis of major clinical trials. J Am Coll Cardiol. 2003;41(9):1529–38.
71. Exner DV, Dries DL, Domanski MJ, Cohn JN. Lesser response to angiotensin converting enzyme inhibitor therapy in black as compared to white patients with left ventricular dysfunc-tion. N Engl J Med. 2001;344(18):1351–7.
72. Gibbs CR, Lip GY, Beevers DG. Angioedema due to ACE inhibitors: increased risk in patients of African origin. Br J Clin Pharmacol. 1999;48(6):861–5.
73. Deswal A, Petersen NJ, Souchek J, Ashton CM, Wray NP. Impact of race on health-care utilization and outcomes in veterans with congestive heart failure. J Am Coll Cardiol. 2004;43(5):778–84.
74. Dries DL, Exner DV, Gersh BJ, Cooper HA, Carson PE, Domanski MJ. Racial differences in the outcome of left ventricular dysfunction. N Engl J Med. 1999;340(8):609–16. Erratum in: N Engl J Med. 1999;341(4):298
75. Taylor AL, Ziesche S, Yancy C, Carson P, D'Agostino R, Ferdinand K, Taylor M, African-American Heart Failure Trial Investigators, et al. Combination of isosorbide dinitrate and hydralazine in blacks with heart failure. N Engl J Med. 2004;351(20):2049–57.
76. Hunt SA, Abraham WT, Chin MH, Feldman AM, Francis GS, Ganiats TG, American College of Cardiology; American Heart Association Task Force on Practice Guidelines; American College of Chest Physicians; International Society for Heart and Lung Transplantation; Heart

Rhythm Society, et al. ACC/AHA 2005 guideline update for the diagnosis and management of chronic heart failure in the adult. Circulation. 2005;112(12):e154–235.

77. Heart Failure Society of America. HFSA 2006 comprehensive heart failure practice guideline. J Card Fail. 2006;12(a):e1–2.

78. Fonarow GC, Yancy CW, Hernandez AF, Peterson ED, Spertus JA, Heidenreich PA. Potential impact of optimal implementation of evidence-based heart failure therapies on mortality. Am Heart J. 2011;161(6):1024–30.e3.

79. Wakeman SE, Barnett ML. Primary care and the opioid crisis - buprenorphine myths and realities. N Engl J Med. 2018;379(1):1–4.

80. Saloner B, Stoller KB, Alexander GC. Moving addiction care to the mainstream—improving the quality of buprenorphine treatment. N Engl J Med. 2018;379(1):4–6.

81. Scruggs AE. Sharp rise in African American opioid overdoses has Cleveland officials worried. The Washington Post. 9 Jun 2017.

82. Katz J, Goodnough A. The opioid crisis is getting worse, particularly for black Americans. The New York Times. 22 Dec 2017.

83. Volkow ND, Collins FS. The role of science in addressing the opioid crisis. N Engl J Med. 2017;377(4):391–4.

84. National Institutes of Health. NIH HEAL Initiative. https://www.nih.gov/research-training/medical-research-initiatives/heal-initiative. Accessed 13 Sep 2019.

85. Wood E. Strategies for reducing opioid-overdose deaths - lessons from Canada. N Engl J Med. 2018;378(17):1565–7.

86. Centers for Disease Control and Prevention. HIV Surveillance Report, 2016. Vol. 28. http://www.cdc.gov/hiv/library/reports/hiv-surveillance.html. Published Nov 2017. Accessed 13 Sep 2019.

87. Epstein JE. Altered conditions: disease, medicine, and storytelling. London/New York: Routledge; 1995. p. 18.

88. Nance RM, Delaney JAC, Simoni JM, Wilson IB, Myer KH, Whitney BM, et al. HIV viral suppression trends over time among HIV-infected patients receiving care in the United States, 1997 to 2015. A cohort study. Ann Intern Med. 2018;169(6):376–84.

89. Thigpen MC, Kebaabetswe PM, Paxton LA, Smith DK, Rose CE, Segolodi TM, TDF2 Study Group. Antiretroviral preexposure prophylaxis for heterosexual HIV transmission in Botswana. N Engl J Med. 2012;367(5):423–34.

90. U.S. Department of Health and Human Services. AIDS info. FDA approves first drug for reducing the risk of sexually acquired HIV infection. 16 Jul 2012. Washington, DC. http://www.fda.gov/NewsEvents/Newsroom/PressAnnouncements/ucm312210.htm. Accessed 13 Sep 2019.

91. Grohskopf LA, Chillag KL, Gvetadze R, Liu AY, Thompson M, Mayer KH, et al. Randomized trial of clinical safety of daily oral tenofovir disoproxil fumarate among HIV uninfected men who have sex with men in the United States. J Acquir Immune Defic Syndr. 2013;64(1):79–86.

92. Centers for Disease Control and Prevention. HIV Surveillance Report, 2015. Vol. 27. https://www.cdc.gov/hiv/pdf/library/reports/surveillance/cdc-hiv-surveillance-report-2015-vol-27.pdf. Accessed Published Nov 2016. Accessed 13 Sep 2019.

93. Bush S, Magnuson D, Rawlings MK, Hawkins T, McCallister S, Mera Giler R. Racial characteristics of FTC/TDF for pre-exposure prophylaxis (PrEP) users in the US (abstract 2651). ASM Microbe 2016/ ICAAC 2016. Boston, MA. 16–20 Jun 2016.

94. Kwakwa HA, Bessias S, Sturgis D, Walton G, Wahome R, Gaye O, Jackson M. Engaging United States black communities in HIV pre-exposure prophylaxis: analysis of a PrEP engagement cascade. J Natl Med Assoc. 2018;110(5):480–5.

95. Albeck-Ripka L. How Australia could almost eradicate HIV transmissions. The New York Times. 10 Jul 2019.

Profiles in Courage: African American Medical Pioneers in the United States—The Earliest Black Practitioners

2

Introduction

We begin this chapter with a description of some of the most unusual people ever to practice the art of medicine. These are the *slave doctors* who were largely untrained except in some cases by their slave masters who were physicians themselves. Although still in bondage, they demonstrated unusual medical and surgical skills which prompted their masters to allow them to treat their fellow slaves, especially in emergency situations. Some of them were actually apprenticed to their masters and, after completion of their training, were permitted to establish formal practices, ultimately earning enough to purchase their freedom.

These early black practitioners gave rise to formally trained physicians who struggled to carry on the tradition of treating their own people against very difficult odds. Eventually, a group of more sophisticated but no less dedicated African American doctors evolved who were committed not only to helping their people survive clinically but also to establishing a footprint of educational, academic, and scholastic excellence that endures to this day. This is the story of the emergence, education, and evolution of the black physician from the time he rose up during slavery through the throes and agony of the Civil War and Reconstruction and progressed into the postwar Jim Crow era and beyond. It is truly a story of triumph over adversity that is one of the most poignant that this nation has ever seen.

The Earliest Black Medical Practitioners

The skills possessed by the practitioners and the treatments that they applied to their subjects were based in folk and herbal medicine derived from their African heritage and culture. An excellent book that provides some account of how these forms of medicine evolved, which is based on oral histories passed down through the generations, is *Black Folk Medicine* by Wilbur H. Watson [1].

© Springer Nature Switzerland AG 2020
R. A. Williams, *Blacks in Medicine*, https://doi.org/10.1007/978-3-030-41960-8_2

It is certainly known that "witch doctors" prevailed in Africa [2] and that this form of treatment transitioned to America on the slave boats. Most likely, the slaves preferred to be treated by their own practitioners according to their own long-established traditional methods proven over the centuries in their homelands, spiritual healing practices that they trusted. There is some evidence that preventive measures were also used such as certain potions, foods, bark, grasses, and other substances that were ingested, worn on the body, or placed in the clothing to ward off evil spirits. One can envision a shaman, priest, witch doctor, or some type of designated medical potentate administering treatments to his subjects, usually in a ritualistic fashion designed to cast out whatever evil demons may have possessed the victim who might be manifesting any type of physical or mental ailment, ranging from fever, convulsions, hemorrhage, and hallucinations to paralysis, tremors, stupor, and beyond.

Voodoo, called *hoodoo* by blacks, was a form of folk medicine used by slave practitioners in certain areas of the country such as Louisiana, Texas, Arkansas, and other parts of the Deep South. Wilbert C. Jordan, MD, a contemporary Harvard-trained infectious disease expert at UCLA, grew up in a voodoo medicine environment in Arkansas and wrote a chapter about his experiences and his in-depth knowledge of the subject in *The Textbook of Black-Related Diseases* [3]. Dr. Jordan stated that his grandmother, who was a voodoo high priestess, used certain roots, herbs, potions, and objects such as voodoo dolls to treat particular conditions that were afflicting the subject. He also provided details of how common conditions such as stomach pains were treated with sugar cubes coated with kerosene and poultices that were prescribed to be worn by victims of pneumonia. Some of these practices endure to this day, especially among Haitian immigrant populations in cities such as New York, Newark, N.J., and Miami, Florida.

The late legendary physician Beny Primm (1928–2015) (Fig. 2.1) quoted Ruth Dennis of the Meharry Medical College who gave a speech there on folk medicine practices and beliefs used in the healthcare of blacks. Among the roots, home remedies, and voodoo practices that were used were the following [1]:

- Honey and lemon and whiskey tea—used to handle a cold.
- Warm saltwater—for fever
- Garlic cloves—for blood pressure
- Eucalyptus oil and honey—for colds
- Fat meat and potatoes—for boils
- Raw egg— for boils
- Penny and chewed tobacco—for rusty nail wound
- Strings tied on the leg—for cramps
- Coins, keys—for bleeding nose
- Beer—for prevention of worms
- Turpentine and sugar—to promote healing of open wounds
- Kerosene and sugar—for colds
- Silver dollar and belly band—for protruding navel

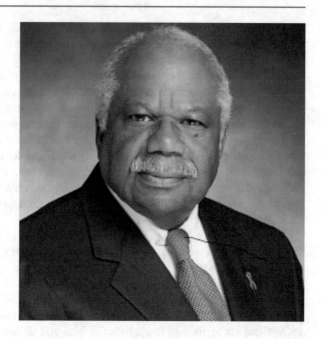

Fig. 2.1 Beny Primm, MD. He was a fierce advocate of focusing attention on the AIDS epidemic in minority communities, and he was also an expert on the use of folk medicine. (Courtesy of www.hiv.gov)

- Mustard seed—for asthma
- Dirt and clay rocks—for headaches
- Standing on head—for headaches

It is important to point out that non-allopathic medical practices are widespread in the United States, and they always have been, not just among the slaves, but among the entire population. Blacks call it *folk medicine*, while whites use the terms *alternative, traditional*, or *complementary* medicine to describe what many consider unorthodox medical practices. All forms have three things in common, no matter what their origin, that distinguish them from allopathic or orthodox medicine or biomedicine: they do not require a prescription; precise dosages are unknown; and there is little or no scientific documentation of their effects. Nonetheless, millions of people have sworn by these holistic remedies for centuries, and the slave doctors at the center of this discussion used substances and methods that likely enjoyed the same popularity. Young [4] has epitomized the basis on which the selection between the different medical choices might be made:

> People everywhere must choose from the several possible courses of action available to them in attempting to treat illness. The question of choice becomes even more significant in non-Western settings where modern medical services, often only recently having become available, represent alternatives to longer established alternative medical practices and native curing specialists. This kind of medical pluralism is common in countries of the Third World, particularly in their rural communities. People in these settings have an especially varied set of options and must regularly choose from among two or more distinct systems of medical knowledge and practice in seeking treatment for an illness [4].

The main components of the slave doctors' approach included three practices: purging, bleeding, and the use of emetics. Many times ancillary methods such as the use of leeches to suck poisons from a victim's body might be used, as well as poultices to draw out substances that were suspected of causing fever. Consumption of nonfood substances such as red clay and dirt, called *cachexia Africanus* or pica, was often used, and the well-known practice of eating tree bark of certain types that might contain cinchona, the source of the antimalarial drug quinine, has been well documented [5]. Asafetida, a gum resin of a plant related to parsley, is an example of a folk medicine remedy that was widely used. The foul-smelling substance was put into a scarf and wrapped around children's necks to ward off colds, whooping cough, and a variety of respiratory illnesses. Mustard plasters were also applied to the chest as a treatment for colds (www.motherearthliving.com/health-and-wellness/slave-medicine).

It should also be pointed out that the alternative medical practices used by slave doctors had other antecedents in history; in fact, one might say that *all* medical practices carried out before our modern, contemporary era were somewhat primitive by current standards. Consider the dictums issued by sages including Hippocrates, Paracelsus, Plato, Galen, and other ancients; as we look back on them from our current vantage point, they seem to be crude attempts by medical authorities of those times to heal and to cure as best they could. We should consider the slave doctors in the same light. We must also remember that some of the most effective medicines developed in recent years originated in folk medicine. A perfect example is the development of the heart drug digitalis from the leaves of the foxglove plant (*Digitalis purpurea*) by William Withering (1741–1799) in England in the eighteenth century [6]. It was used to treat dropsy (heart failure) with great success, and at one time it became the principal cardiac medicine utilized by practitioners.

The importance of the folk medicine practitioner and his or her role in applying the healing arts must not be underestimated. For blacks during much of their history in the United States, this was "the only game in town," as the saying goes. There was basically little or no access to "white" medical care, and in any event there was not much trust in white physicians and white hospitals. It must be understood that utilization of folk remedies was not a matter of default but of preference or choice of the familiar and the traditional over something that frankly was perceived as more threatening and disturbing rather than comforting. Besides, blacks had no money to pay the white physician, and the few black physicians who came upon the scene had a hard time making ends meet based on the small amount of revenue that they could generate; many had to terminate their practices because they became impecunious. The practice of bartering was heavily used, in which the physician was paid in trade for his services.

Midwives were also used heavily in the South [7]. They often worked in conjunction with physicians or practiced on their own. Sometimes a midwife owned the only hospital in town where blacks could receive treatment or where black physicians could practice. Schools of midwifery were also established in an attempt to raise the standard of treatment dispensed by these women. Many times, a midwife would be called to deliver a black mother's baby, rather than a physician, who was more expensive and less available; the midwife yielded to the physician if the pregnancy was complicated, such as a breech presentation. During the nineteenth century, men began to practice midwifery, and with the development of the obstetrical forceps, they became dominant in this discipline presumably because they could exert more strength in extracting the baby, especially in difficult situations. This trend formed the basis of modern obstetrics. Although midwifery is still practiced in the United States, it is not as available as it once was, mainly because of restrictions imposed by many Southern counties and the imposition of public health regulations. Today, midwives are qualified and certified professionals who are well trained to perform the duties of assisting a pregnant woman in delivering her baby. Another category of assistant is the doula (derived from the ancient Greek word doule', meaning a female who helps). She provides non-medical physical and emotional support to the woman in the prenatal, birthing, or postnatal period.

Another unorthodox medical practitioner in the black community was the "drug store doctor," who was found especially in New Orleans. He operated in the back rooms of drug stores or pharmacies and dispensed folk remedies to clients for a variety of ills. There were also spiritual practitioners, who sometimes were located in the back rooms of grocery stores in small Southern towns, who gave advice and provided services for interpersonal problems of various sorts. Unfortunately, some of these operators performed abortions and other illicit procedures on their uneducated customers, often with deadly results. This was the downside of unorthodox medical practices, which preyed upon the desperate circumstances of many in the black community. It should be pointed out that not all folk medicine practice was characterized by this type of predatory behavior.

It is well documented that there was and still is a competition between folk or traditional medicine, as practiced by early black healthcare providers and biomedical practitioners. With all due respect that must be given to biomedical science in combatting disease and making the United States the preeminent world leader in medicine, we must nonetheless recognize the critical role that traditional medicine has played in the well-being and, indeed, the very survival of blacks who arguably may not have endured without it. One might say that this type of medical practice was the linchpin or connector between slavery and modern times; it provided the means by which black people were able to keep on going forward despite terrible health conditions and environmental circumstances that were imposed upon them.

As time went on, the two approaches to healthcare delivery came closer together but have never been truly merged. Allopathic medicine has tended to view folk medicine with some skepticism and even derision, but more recently the development of *integrative* and *complementary* medicine, also called *alternative medicine*, has provided more respect for the latter, especially since the National Institutes of Health has been investigating the subject since 1991 and has now established the National Center for Complementary and Integrative Health (https://nccih.nih.gov/).

The Slave Doctors of America

The first of the early slave doctors was not a resident of the South but was actually enslaved to the eminent Boston Puritan minister and scientist Cotton Mather. He is memorialized by only one name, Onesimus, and he came to prominence because of his brilliant work in attempting to develop a cure for smallpox, which was endemic in Massachusetts during the time of his servitude. Onesimus developed an inoculation against smallpox that was successfully used by Dr. Zabdiel Boylston in combating an epidemic in Boston in 1721 [8]. Paradoxically, some white residents of Boston rebelled and stormed Dr. Boylston's home when they found out that the technique had been developed by a black slave. Onesimus's inoculation technique no doubt was the inspiration for the development of vaccination against smallpox by Jenner, who was the one memorialized in history. As Sir Francis Galton stated, "…in science, credit goes to the man who convinces the world, not to the man to whom the idea first occurs." Galton emphatically denied that Jenner initiated the concept of inoculation as a protection against smallpox, stating that the practice had been used successfully in England before Jenner, who was inoculated himself as a boy [9]. Galton gave credit for the practice to others who predated Jenner, including Cotton Mather, who had credited his slave Onesimus [10]. As Mather himself told the story [11]:

> I had from a servant of my own an account of its being practiced in Africa. Enquiring of my Negro man, Onesimus, who is a pretty intelligent fellow, whether he ever had the smallpox, he answered both yes and no; and then he told me that he had undergone an operation, which had given him something of the smallpox and would forever preserve him from it.…He described the operation to me and showed me in his arm the scar which it had left upon him …

Primus, another slave in New England, learned surgery from his master who was a surgeon and took over the physician's practice when he died, becoming extraordinarily successful. He pioneered in the treatment of rabies [12].

Papan, a Virginian slave, was so proficient in developing cures for skin and venereal diseases that he was freed by the Virginia Legislature in 1729 after purchasing him from his master "as a reward for so useful a discovery which may be of great benefit to mankind" [8].

Caesar, a slave in South Carolina, had an extensive knowledge of herbs and roots, which he used to treat a variety of diseases. He wrote the first medical publication by an African American, on a remedy for snakebite, which was published by the *Massachusetts Magazine* in 1792 [8].The South Carolina Assembly not only purchased his freedom in 1792, they also gave him a lifetime annuity of $500, a substantial amount at the time.

James Durham or Derham was a slave originally owned by Philadelphia physician John Kearsley, Jr., who taught him medicine. After his owner's death, he was purchased by and apprenticed to three other doctors who continued to teach medicine to him. Eventually, he was purchased by Dr. Robert Dove of New Orleans, from whom he purchased his freedom. He became one of the leading physicians in New Orleans in the late 1700s. So great was his fame and reputation that the legendary Dr. Benjamin Rush met with him and spoke about him with consummate praise:

I have conversed with him upon most of the acute and epidemic diseases of the country
Where he lives, and was pleased to find him perfectly acquainted with the modern
Simple mode of practice in those diseases. I expected to have suggested some new
medicines to him, but he suggested many more to me [13].

However, because of jealousy and the fact that he lacked formal training in medicine, he did not receive patient referrals from his white peers sufficient to sustain his practice. He eventually disappeared from the scene in 1802 and was lost to history.

The First Licensed Black Physicians in America

Although he was of Dutch origin, Dr. Lucas Santomee is generally recognized as the first black physician to practice in the United States. Educated in Holland, he practiced in New York, or New Amsterdam, during the Colonial Period (circa 1600) [8].

James McCune Smith, MD (1813–1865) (Fig. 2.2), was born in New York City of a free mother and a father who was an ex-slave and a successful merchant. Denied admission to institutions of higher learning in the United States, he entered the University of Glasgow, Scotland, in 1832. He is credited with being the first black person to graduate from *any* medical school, receiving three degrees in Glasgow: the BA, the MA, and the MD (1837); but he received no degrees from a school in the United States. Dr. Smith carried on a highly respected and financially successful medical practice in New York City where most of his patients were white. He was also a noted abolitionist [14].

John David Peck, MD, also known as David Jones Peck, was the first black graduate of an American medical school (Rush Medical School, 1847), 10 years after Dr. James McCune Smith had completed his matriculation. He was not as successful in carrying on a viable medical practice as Dr. Smith, mainly because the black patients among whom he practiced could not afford to pay him. To make

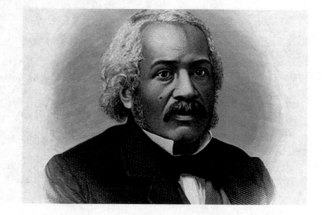

Fig. 2.2 James McCune Smith, MD. (Engraving by Patrick H. Reason. From *Recollections of Seventy Years* by Daniel Alexander Payne [1811–1893], published in 1888. This work is in the public domain in its country of origin and other countries and areas where the copyright term is the author's life plus 70 years or less)

ends meet, he and other early black physicians were forced to do other jobs, which of course made it impossible to focus solely on medicine. Dr. Peck, a protégé of Dr. Martin Robison Delaney, became disillusioned with the prospects of having a successful medical practice as a black doctor in America, and he eventually emigrated to Nicaragua where he joined Dr. Martin Robison Delaney in setting up a new town in an attempt to establish a Negro republic in Latin America. He was killed in 1855 in a military battle there [15].

It was during the Civil War that one saw the emergence of a significant number of black physicians in America. Several, 13 in all, served in the Union Army Medical Corps as physicians and surgeons. They included John Van Surly DeGrasse, MD (1825–1868) (Fig. 2.3); Anderson Ruffin Abbott, MD (1837–1913) (Fig. 2.4), a

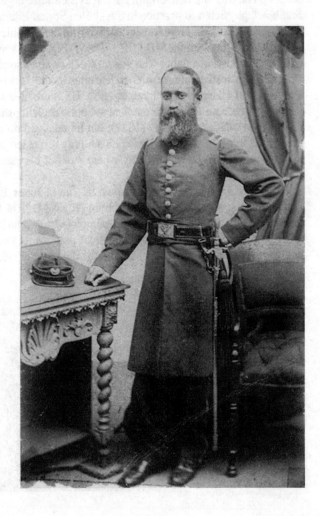

Fig. 2.3 John Van Surly DeGrasse, MD [standing with sword], carte de visite taken by James Wallace Black (Boston, Mass.), circa 1861–1862. (From the original in the DeGrasse-Howard photographs, Massachusetts Historical Society, Boston, Massachusetts)

Fig. 2.4 Anderson Ruffin Abbott, MD. (Courtesy Toronto Public Library; public domain. This work is in the public domain in the US because it was published (or registered with the US Copyright Office) before 1 January 1924)

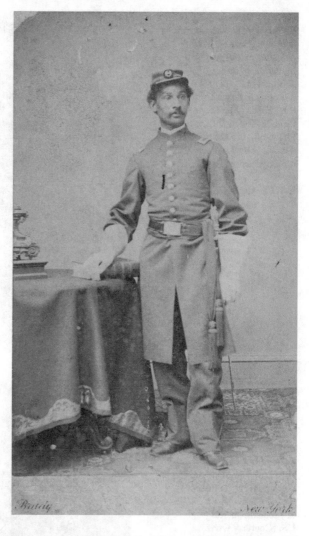

graduate of Toronto Medical School; Charles B. Purvis, MD (1842–1929) (Fig. 2.5); and William P. Powell, Jr., MD, who served as a surgeon in the Union Army. Two of the more prominent individuals were Alexander T. Augusta, MD (1825–1890) (Fig. 2.6), an Army physician who later served as Superintendent of Freedmen's Hospital in Washington, DC, during the 1860s, and Martin Robison Delaney, MD (1812–1885) (Fig. 2.7), who attended Harvard Medical School as the first black student in 1850. He was not to finish Harvard because he and two other blacks, Daniel Laing, Jr., and Isaac H. Snowden, were boycotted by fellow students and were summarily expelled by the famous Dean Oliver Wendell Holmes after less

Fig. 2.5 Charles
B. Purvis, MD, was one of
the founders of Howard
University College of
Medicine. (Courtesy
Schomburg Center for
Research in Black Culture/
New York Public Library/
Science Photo Library.
This work is in the public
domain in the US because
it was published [or
registered with the
U.S. Copyright Office]
before 1 January 1924)

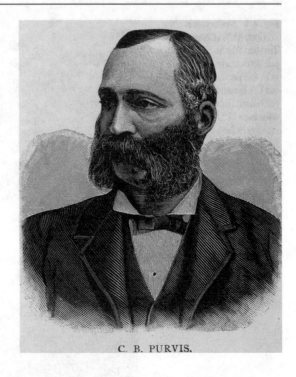

C. B. PURVIS.

Fig. 2.6 Alexander
T. Augusta, MD, was the
highest ranking African
American in the Union
Army (Lt. Colonel), the
first black to head a
hospital (Freedmen's
Hospital), and the first
black medical professor at
Howard University College
of Medicine in the
US. (Courtesy www.
blackpast.org. Public
Domain Mark 1.0)

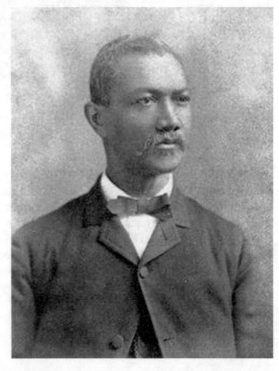

Fig. 2.7 Martin Robison Delany, MD, was one of the first blacks to attend Harvard Medical School, a prominent African American newspaper editor, and the first African American major in the US Army. (From original in the Civil War Photograph Collection, RG 98s of the U.S. Army Heritage and Education Center, Carlisle, PA. This media file is in the public domain in the US. This applies to US works where the copyright has expired, often because its first publication occurred prior to 1 January 1924 and if not then due to lack of notice or renewal)

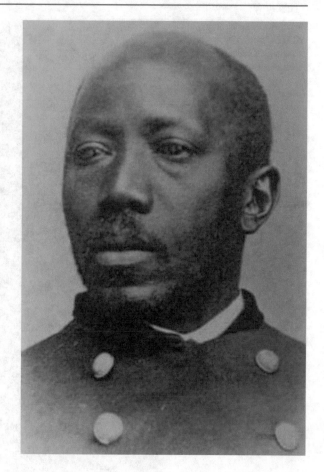

than 2 years of matriculation. The reason for their expulsion, as explained by Dean Holmes, was that "…the intermixing of the black and white races in their lecture rooms is distasteful to a large portion of the class and injurious to the interests of the school" [16]. He was forced to complete his medical training through apprenticeship or preceptorship, following which he entered the Union Army and rose to the rank of Major. Incidentally, Harvard Medical School did not graduate its first black physician until almost 20 years after Delaney, Laing, and Snowden were expelled; Edwin C.J.T. Howard received the MD degree from Harvard in 1869.

Other black physicians who practiced during this period were Dr. Thomas J. White, who was a graduate of Bowdoin College in Maine along with Dr. DeGrasse; Peter W. Ray, MD (1825–1906) (Fig. 2.8), who graduated in1850 from Castleton Medical College in Vermont and practiced in New York City; Edwin C. Howard, MD (1846–1912) (Fig. 2.9), and Frederick Douglass Stubbs, MD (1906–1947) (Fig. 2.10) [17], both of whom graduated from Harvard Medical School and later co-founded Mercy-Douglass Hospital in Philadelphia; and John Sweat Rock, MD,

Fig. 2.8   Peter W. Ray,
MD (1825–1906).
(Courtesy Black Gotham
Archives, from original in
the New York Public
Library)

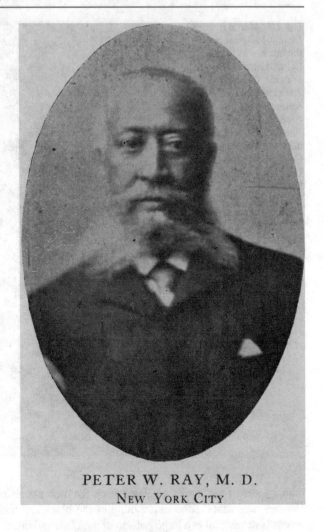

PETER W. RAY, M. D.
NEW YORK CITY

DDS, JD (1825–1866) (Fig. 2.11), who practiced in Boston in the 1850s as a physician and a dentist. He was also the first black person to be admitted to the bar of the US Supreme Court. Another African American physician of note during the late nineteenth century was Daniel Hale Williams, MD (1856–1931) (Fig. 2.12), who founded Provident Hospital in Chicago, the first black-owned hospital in America, and who is credited with performing the first operation on the living human heart in 1893, a pericardiotomy, on a stabbing victim. Dr. Williams was also one of the founders of the National Medical Association in 1895.

Indeed, the last half of the nineteenth century, and particularly after 1868, was a period of relatively great growth of the numbers of blacks in the health profession. Spurred mainly by a determination to care for themselves and to establish institutions of medical and nursing training, they started their own hospitals, schools of nursing, and even medical schools.

Fig. 2.9 Edwin
C. Howard, MD (circa
1893). Schillare
(Northampton,
Massachusetts). University
Photograph Collection (RG
130). (Special Collections
and University Archives,
University of
Massachusetts Amherst
Libraries, with permission)

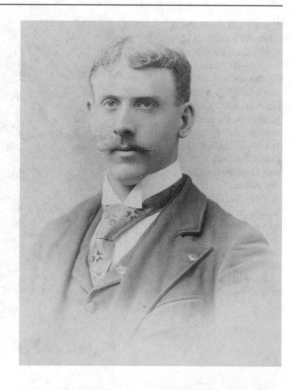

Fig. 2.10 Frederick
Douglass Stubbs, MD
(1906–1947). (Courtesy of
the *Journal of the National
Medical Association* and
H. Gordon Fleming on
behalf of the
Stubbs family)

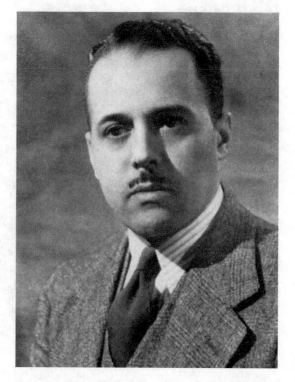

Fig. 2.11 John Sweat Rock, MD, DDS, JD, was a physician, dentist, and lawyer who practiced in Boston and was admitted to the Massachusetts Bar. (John H. Rock, Colored Counselor. By Richards, Philadelphia. *Harper's Weekly* 25 February 1854. Public Domain. https://commons.wikimedia.org/w/index.php?curid=8716216. This work is in the public domain in its country of origin and other countries and areas where the copyright term is the author's life plus 70 years or less)

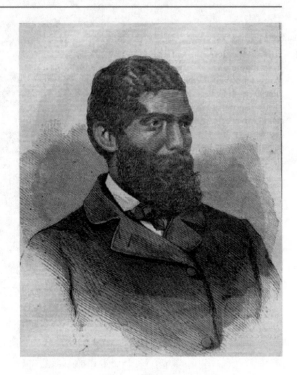

Fig. 2.12 Daniel Hale Williams, MD. (Courtesy National Library of Medicine Digital Collection. NLM Unique ID:101448033)

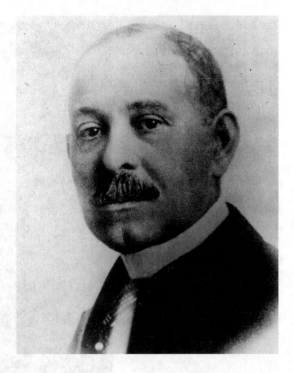

It should be noted that black women had a more difficult time entering into medicine than black men did; one might say that they suffered double discrimination, i.e., race and gender. As mentioned above, Dr. John David Peck was the first black male to graduate from an American medical school, in 1847. It was not until 1864 that the first black woman physician, Rebecca Lee Crumpler, MD (1831–1895), earned her medical degree from the New England Female Medical College located in Boston. Born in Delaware and raised in Philadelphia, she practiced briefly in Boston after receiving a degree of "doctress" of medicine as the first and only black woman to graduate from that institution. After the Civil War ended in 1865, she moved to Richmond, Virginia, where she served through the Freedmen's Bureau as a medical missionary for freed slaves who had no other source of medical care. She published one of the earliest medical books by a black person, entitled *A Book of Medical Discourses*, in 1883 about her experiences in providing care for the indigent [18]. Subsequent black women medical graduates were few and far between. After Dr. Rebecca Lee Crumpler came Dr. Rebecca Cole, who graduated from Women's Medical College of Pennsylvania in 1867, and then Dr. Susan Maria Smith McKinney Steward, who received her degree from New York Medical College and Hospital for Women in 1870. Their admission into the medical profession occurred roughly at the same time that efforts began to eliminate the suppression of women in American society and to secure equal rights for them in all fields of endeavor.

Some other notable black physicians who were pioneers in medicine in the first half of the twentieth century were:

William Augustus Hinton, MD (1883–1959), was the first black professor at Harvard Medical School. He wrote the first medical book authored by an African American physician, *Syphilis and its Treatment* (1936), and pioneered the Hinton test for syphilis (Fig. 2.13).

Charles R. Drew, MD (1904–1950) (Fig. 2.14), attended Amherst and subsequently entered McGill University in Quebec, Canada, to study medicine, graduating in 1933 as a member of the Alpha Omega Alpha scholastic medical society [19]. After a brief period serving on the faculty of Howard University and of Freedmen's Hospital in the Department of Surgery, he did graduate work in surgery at Columbia University in New York City where he earned a Doctor of Science in Surgery. Later, working under a Rockefeller Fellowship, he earned a Doctor of Science in Medicine while doing rigorous research on "banked blood," which was concerned with techniques of blood preservation. He also started the Bloodmobile system that provided transportation of blood to needed locations and also facilitated donation and collection of blood. In 1940, Dr. Drew was recruited to be the medical director of a program called Blood for Britain, in which he oversaw the testing, collection, and transportation of large quantities of blood plasma for use in the United Kingdom during World War II. The program was enormously successful, and in 1941 Dr. Drew was appointed to head the first American Red Cross Blood Bank. However, he resigned from this post in 1942 after the armed forces ruled that blood collected from African Americans would have to be stored separately from that of whites. He then became the first black examiner for the American Board of Surgery, and in 1942 he returned to Howard University

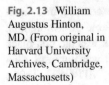
Fig. 2.13 William
Augustus Hinton,
MD. (From original in
Harvard University
Archives, Cambridge,
Massachusetts)

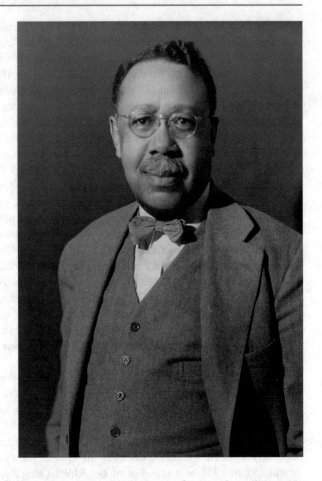

and Freedmen's Hospital, becoming a surgeon and a professor of medicine. He
received numerous accolades and honors in recognition of his brilliant research
and public service, including the Spingarn Medal from the National Association
for the Advancement of Colored People (NAACP). In 1950, during a road trip to
Tuskegee Institute in Alabama, he died at age 45 from injuries in an automobile
accident. He memorably said that "Excellence of performance will transcend arti-
ficial barriers created by man." His legacy has been perpetuated in the form of the
Charles R. Drew University of Medicine and Science, the third historically black
college or university (HBCU) medical school after Howard and Meharry, founded
in 1966 in Watts, California.

In 1940 Louis T. Wright, MD (1891–1952) (Fig. 2.15), was also awarded of
the NAACP's Spingarn Medal in recognition of his political activism as well as
for his medical expertise. His parents were former slaves [20, 21]. He was born in
LaGrange, Georgia, and went on to receive a BA from Clark University in Atlanta
and an MD degree from Harvard Medical School, where he began his social activism by joining protests and picketing against D.W. Griffith's racist film, *Birth of a*

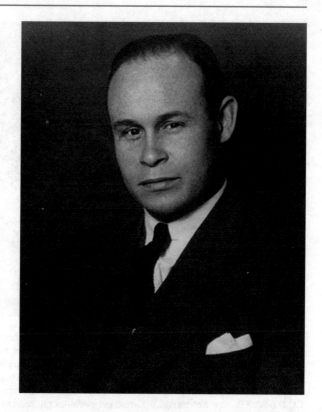

Fig. 2.14 Charles R. Drew, MD. The former Chairman of Surgery at Howard University College of Medicine, his research and innovations in blood banking saved thousands of lives in World War II. (Associated Photographic Services, Inc. National Library of Medicine: http://profiles.nlm.nih.gov/ps/retrieve/ResourceMetadata/BGBBCT: Year supplied: ca. 1949. From original repository: Howard University. Moorland-Spingarn Research Center. Charles R. Drew Papers, PD-US, https://en.wikipedia.org/w/index.php?curid=47837720)

Nation. Despite the time that he lost from his medical studies, he still finished fourth in his graduating class from Harvard in 1915. He then joined the US Army and served with the rank of Captain as a physician in France during World War I where he helped to save many lives and suffered battlefield injuries himself, for which he was decorated with the Purple Heart. Upon returning from the war, he moved to New York City where he joined the staff as the first black surgeon at Harlem Hospital in 1919, which at that time was in bad repair. He almost singlehandedly got the hospital renovated, had the professional staff upgraded, raised the patient care standards of the hospital, and moved it into national eminence.

At the same time, he continued to work with the NAACP and protested against racism in medicine, including the widespread notion that blacks were more prone to develop and harbor syphilis and other infectious diseases because they possessed biological and constitutional weaknesses that made them more vulnerable to such diseases. He also developed the intradermal injection vaccination technique and was one of the earliest black members of the American College of Surgeons. He established the Harlem Hospital Cancer Research Foundation, became the first to conduct research on the new drug chlortetracycline (trade name Aureomycin), and developed an expertise in the treatment of head injuries. He served as Director of Surgery and as President of the Medical Board until 1949 when he retired from Harlem Hospital. He died from tuberculosis in New York City at the age of 61.

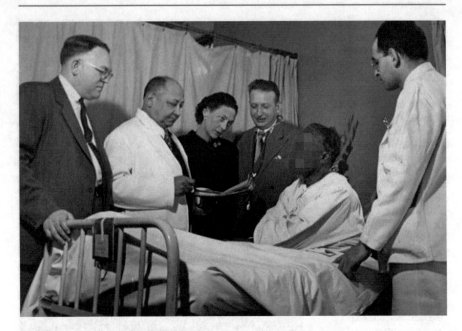

Fig. 2.15 Louis T. Wright, MD, and colleagues at patient bedside, Harlem Hospital, New York, NY. From left to right: Dr. Lyndon M. Hill, Dr. Louis T. Wright, Dr. Myra Logan, Dr. Aaron Prigot, unidentified African American woman patient, and unidentified hospital employee. (By Joe Covello (for Black Star). From original in Louis Tompkins Wright papers, 1879, 1898, 1909–1997. H MS c56. Harvard Medical Library, Francis A. Countway Library of Medicine, Boston, Mass., CC BY-SA 3.0, https://commons.wikimedia.org/w/index.php?curid=46672800)

More Recent Black Medical Trailblazers

Samuel L. Kountz, MD (1930–1981) (Fig. 2.16), grandson of a woman born into slavery and son of a Baptist minister, was the first black to enter the University of Arkansas Medical School at Little Rock. He was first associated with the University of California School of Medicine in San Francisco and Stanford Medical Center, where he did animal experiments in kidney transplantation. He performed the first successful kidney transplant using a donor and a recipient who were not identical twins in 1961, thus opening up renal transplantation to thousands of kidney disease victims, a procedure that literally saved their lives. He discovered that methylprednisolone in large doses could prevent acute rejection of a transplanted kidney. That steroid was used for many years to manage kidney transplant patients. With other researchers he developed the prototype of a machine that is now able to preserve kidneys for up to 50 hours from the time

Fig. 2.16 Samuel
L. Kountz,
MD. (Photograph courtesy
of the University of
California at San Francisco
Archives and Special
Collections, Photograph
Collection, Portraits, Dr.
Samuel L. Kountz)

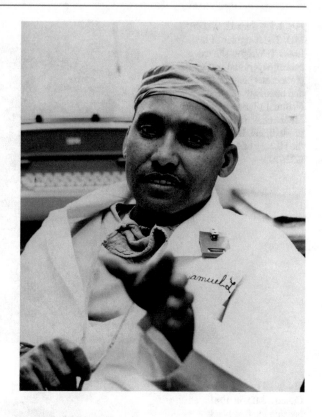

they are removed from the donor's body. The machine is used worldwide and is named the Belzer kidney perfusion machine in honor of Dr. Kountz's partner, Dr. Folkert O. Belzer. He also advanced tissue typing tests to improve the results of kidney transplantation. Dr. Kountz moved across country to become head of surgery at the SUNY Downstate Medical Center in Brooklyn. He told friends that he moved to Brooklyn to improve medical care for the black community. He performed 500 kidney transplants prior to his tragic illness and death. Following a trip to South Africa as a visiting professor in 1977, he incurred a disease that was never diagnosed but left him brain-damaged and in home care for the remainder of his life [22].

This chapter features just a few of the African American women who were pioneers in medicine, including Jane C. Wright, MD (1919–2013) (Fig. 2.17); Alexa Irene Canady, MD (1950–) (Fig. 2.18); Marilyn Hughes Gaston, MD (1939–) (Fig. 2.19); Patricia Era Bath, MD (1942–2019) (Fig. 2.20); and Mae Jemison, MD (1956–) (Fig. 2.21). They represent the black female trailblazers who are too numerous to depict here, but we salute all of them for their courage and tenacity.

Fig. 2.17 Jane C. Wright, MD. The daughter of Dr. Louis T. Wright, she was a cancer expert and was a pioneer in chemotherapy and oncology. (Courtesy National Library of Medicine National Library of Medicine, Images from the History of Medicine, B026209)

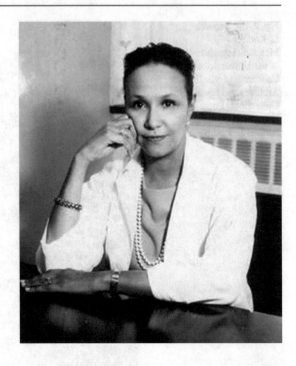

Fig. 2.18 Alexa Irene Canady, MD, in 1981 became the first black neurosurgeon in the United States. Educated at the University of Michigan, she served as Chief of Neurosurgery at Children's Hospital of Michigan. (Courtesy of the National Library of Medicine, Changing the Face of Medicine Exhibition, https://cfmedicine.nlm.nih.gov/physicians/biography_53.html)

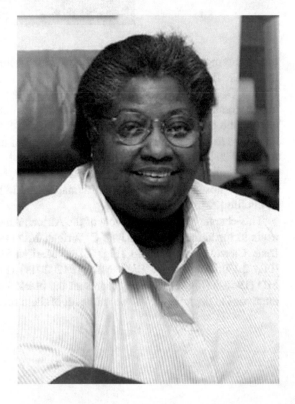

Fig. 2.19 Marilyn Hughes Gaston, MD. Assistant US Surgeon General and Rear Admiral, she was the first African American female director of a public health bureau, the US Department of Health and Human Services Administration (HRSA) Bureau of Primary Health Care. She also conducted very important research which led to screening newborn children for sickle cell anemia for immediate treatment, and she pioneered the use of antibiotics in infants with sickle cell disease which saved hundreds of lives. (Courtesy of the National Library of Medicine, Changing the Face of Medicine Exhibition, https://cfmedicine.nlm.nih.gov/physicians/biography_124.html)

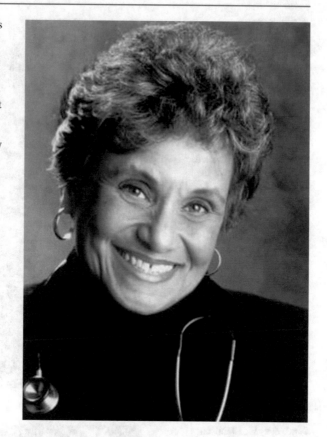

The field of nursing opened up to women at about this time, thanks to the heroic efforts of Florence Nightingale who founded the first school of nursing in 1860. Nursing became an alternative to medicine for many women who were not accepted by medical schools; it became firmly established as a companion to the practice of medicine. Mary Eliza Mahoney, RN (1845–1926), was the first African American professional nurse. She graduated from the New England Hospital for Women and Children School of Nursing in 1879 (Fig. 2.22). Nurses and midwives became essential participants in the delivery of healthcare for blacks, especially in the rural South (Fig. 2.23), and many nursing schools were opened for African American students to pursue the field (Fig. 2.24).

Fig. 2.20 Patricia Era
Bath, MD. An expert in
ophthalmology, she was
the first African American
woman surgeon to serve on
staff at the UCLA Medical
Center and the first to head
an ophthalmology training
program. Her invention of
laser methods to treat eye
disease is said to have led
to the development of the
Lasik® technique.
(Courtesy of the National
Library of Medicine,
Changing the Face of
Medicine Exhibition,
https://cfmedicine.nlm.nih.
gov/physicians/
biography_26.html)

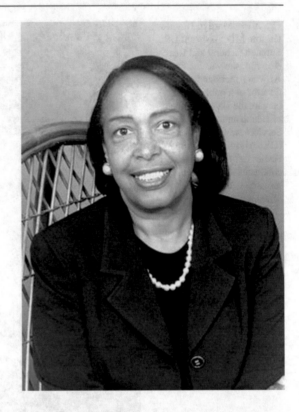

Fig. 2.21 Mae Jemison,
MD. In 1992, she literally
flew into history by
becoming the first black
female astronaut to
complete a mission in
space. (Courtesy of
Johnson Space Center of
the United States National
Aeronautics and Space
Administration (NASA),
Photo ID: S92-40463)

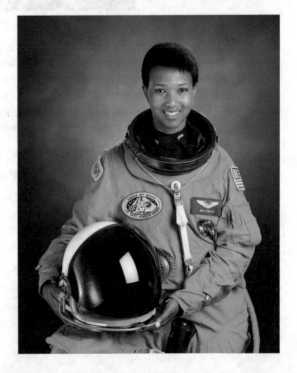

Fig. 2.22 Mary Eliza Mahoney, RN (Unknown photographer. http://www.hcrhealth.com/content/our-community/blog/black-history-month-profile-mary-eliza-mahoney and as appears on the cover of Mary Eliza Mahoney, Public Domain, https://commons.wikimedia.org/w/index.php?curid=20285831)

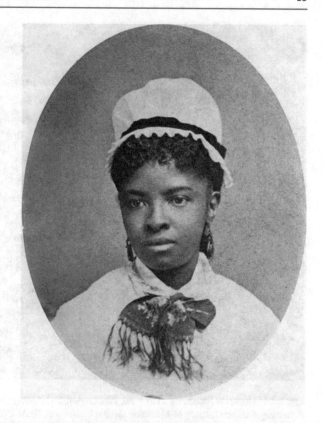

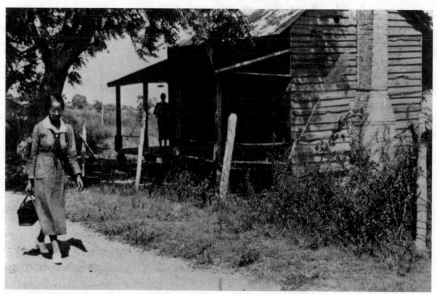

Fig. 2.23 A black nurse visiting a rural house in the 1920s. Nurses and midwives carried a large part of the healthcare burden in the rural South. (Courtesy National Library of Medicine Digital Collection. NLM Unique ID:101447749)

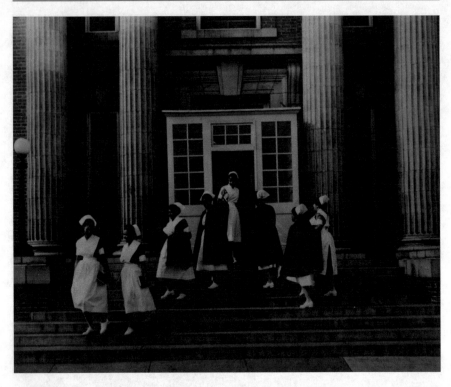

Fig. 2.24 Nurses at Freedmen's Hospital, Washington, DC. Source: National Library of Medicine. (Courtesy National Library of Medicine Digital Collection. NLM Unique ID:101446067)

Conclusion

This presentation on black pioneers in medicine would not be complete without mentioning the legendary Vivien Theodore Thomas (1910–1985) [23] (Fig. 2.25), who was not a classically trained physician but who nevertheless succeeded as the black surgical assistant who helped to devise the famous "blue baby" operation at The Johns Hopkins Hospital in Baltimore. He was later given an honorary Doctor of Medical Science degree by the university in recognition of his expertise.

Another black surgeon at that iconic institution who achieved outstanding accomplishments was Levi Watkins, Jr., MD (1944–2015) (Fig. 2.26), a heart surgeon at The Johns Hopkins Hospital who implanted the first cardiac defibrillator (assisted by Vivien Thomas) in a human patient only 7 months after he had finished his surgical training. He was also an ardent civil rights pioneer and crusader for diversity in medicine, having participated in the Montgomery bus boycott as a teenager and volunteered as a part-time driver for Dr. Martin Luther King, Jr., who was his family's pastor. Dr. Watkins was the first black student to enter and graduate from the Vanderbilt University School of Medicine. In an interview with the University of Alabama at Birmingham, whose all-white medical school had denied him admission years earlier, he said: "All my work since the integration of Vanderbilt University

Fig. 2.25 Vivien Theodore Thomas, MD (1910–1985). Working as a surgical assistant at Johns Hopkins Hospital with heart surgeon Dr. Alfred Blaylock and Pediatric Cardiologist Dr. Helen Taussig, he helped to devise the "blue baby" operation to correct the tetralogy of Fallot (http://www.blackpast.org/aah/thomas-vivien-1910-1985, Public Domain, https://commons.wikimedia.org/w/index.php?curid=33457689)

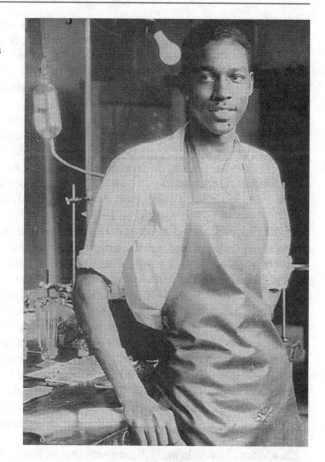

Fig. 2.26 Levi Watkins, Jr., MD. (Kingkongphoto & www.celebrity-photos.com from Laurel Maryland, USA – Dr. Levi Watkins of Hopkins University, CC BY-SA 2.0, https://commons.wikimedia.org/w/index.php?curid=74827761)

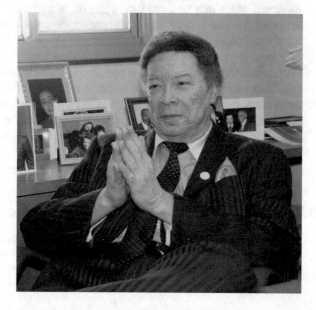

has been about inclusion, equity and opportunity" [24]. Another alumnus of Johns Hopkins, Ben Carson, MD (Benjamin Solomon Carson, Sr.), grew up in Detroit and graduated from Yale and the University of Michigan Medical School. Carson was the Director of Pediatric Neurosurgery at The Johns Hopkins Hospital from 1984 until his retirement in 2013, and was renowned for performing the first successful separation of infant twins conjoined at the head [25].

This brief review of folk medicine, early traditional medical practices, slave doctors, the first blacks to practice medicine, and black medical pioneers is meant to serve as an entrée to the involvement of blacks in medicine on a larger, more orthodox scale. It is a prelude to the current black medical scene, and one should understand the fact that the manner in which current black health professionals evolved derives directly from this background. It also forms the basis for the way that many African American patients view, utilize, and accept physicians, hospitals, clinics, and other aspects of healthcare. It must be recognized that there is a continuum from the past to the present and that unless this connection between past traditional practices and the beliefs that many blacks still have about medicine is recognized, current practitioners may have difficulty reaching black patients and achieving success with their treatments. This is why it is so important to talk to the patient and to find out what he or she thinks about the treatment that the physician proposes to use. Unfortunately, this approach has been used too infrequently by busy physicians. One of the aims of the Affordable Care Act (https://www.hhs.gov/healthcare/about-the-aca/index.html) (aka Obamacare or ACA) is to place the patient at the center of the healthcare universe rather than the physician and to involve the patient as a partner in his or her care. The initiation of the Patient-Centered Outcomes Research Institute (https://www.pcori.org/) (PCORI), which is a quasi-government agency operating for the public benefit created under the Affordable Care Act (ACA or Obamacare), is designed to do exactly that.

In addition, the development of a renewed interest in complementary and alternative medicine, which may be considered offshoots of traditional medical practices, is also important because it takes into consideration the value that this approach to healing has for the public. Because of its significance in the healthcare paradigm for blacks over the centuries, as described above, it must be allowed to take its place alongside of allopathic medicine as an effective, practical, acceptable, and genuine form of medical care. This means that it should be taught in medical schools across the board, and its unorthodox treatments should also be subjected to strict scrutiny and inspected and regulated just as allopathic medicine is. The hope is that this will provide additional features to our great system of healthcare in the US that will benefit all people.

References

1. Watson WH, editor. Black folk medicine: the therapeutic significance of faith and trust. New Brunswick: Transaction; 1984.
2. Lugira AM. African traditional religion. New York: Infobase Publishing; 2009. p. 100.
3. Williams RA. Textbook of black-related diseases. New York: McGraw-Hill; 1975.
4. Young JC. Medical choice in a Mexican village. New Brunswick: Rutgers University Press; 1981. p. 3.

5. Staines HM, Krishna S, editors. Treatment and prevention of malaria: antimalarial drug action, chemistry, and use. Basel: Springer Basel AG; 2012. p. 45.

6. Withering W. An account of the foxglove and some of its medical uses: with practical remarks on dropsy, and other diseases. Birmingham: M. Swinney, 1785. Project Gutenberg Ebook: http://library.umac.mo/ebooks/b2834599x.pdf.

7. Litoff JB. American midwives: 1860 to the present. Westport: Greenwood Press; 1978.

8. Rogers JA. Africa's gift to America: the Afro-American in the making and saving of the United States with new supplement Africa and its potentialities. [Place of publication not identified]: Helga M. Rogers; [2014?] ©1961. p. 224.

9. Wilson DE. Minorities in the medical profession: a historical perspective and analysis of current and future trends. J Natl Med Assoc. 1986;78(3):177–80.

10. Gross CP, Sepkowitz KA. The myth of the medical breakthrough: smallpox, vaccination, and Jenner reconsidered. Int J Infect Dis. 1998;3(1):54–60.

11. Kittredge GL. Some lost works of Cotton Mather. Proc Mass Hist Soc. 1912;45:418–40.

12. Greene LJ. The Negro in colonial New England, 1620–1776. Eastford: Martino Fine Books; 2017.

13. Morais HM. The history of the Negro in medicine. New York: Publishers Co.; 1968.

14. Bousfield MO. An account of physicians of color in the United States. Bull Hist Med. 1945;17:61–84.

15. Cobb WM. Dr. David John Peck: first Negro to graduate from an American medical school. Bull Meico-Chirurgical Soc District of Columbia. 1949;6(2):3.

16. Kennedy R. Introduction. In: Sollers W, Titcomb C, Underwood A, editors. Blacks at Harvard: a documentary history of African-American experience at Harvard and Radcliffe. New York/London: New York University Press; 1993. p. xix.

17. Cobb WM. Frederick Douglass Stubbs, 1906–1947: an appreciation. J Natl Med Assoc. 1948;40(1):24–6.

18. U.S. National Library of Medicine. Dr. Rebecca Lee Crumpler. Changing the face of medicine. https://cfmedicine.nlm.nih.gov/physicians/biography_73.html. Accessed 15 Dec 2019.

19. Yancy AS Sr. The life of Charles R. Drew, MD. In: Organ Jr CH, editor. A century of black surgeons: the USA experience. Norman: Transcript Press; 1987.

20. Low WA, Clift VA. Lewis Tompkins Wright. In: Encyclopedia of black America. New York: DaCapo Press; 1981.

21. Reynolds PP. Dr. Louis T. Wright and the NAACP: pioneers in hospital racial integration. Am J Public Health. 2000;90(6):883–92. https://www.ncbi.nlm.nih.gov/pmc/articles/PMC1446256/pdf/10846505.pdf.

22. Altman LK. Dr. Samuel Kountz, 51, dies; leader in transplant surgery. the New York Times. 24 Dec 1981, Section B, Page 6.

23. Timmermans S. A black technician and blue babies. Soc Stud Sci. 2003;33:197–229.

24. Roberts S. Levi Watkins, 70, dies; pioneering heart surgeon pushed civil rights. New York Times. 16 Apr 2015. https://www.nytimes.com/2015/04/17/health/levi-watkins-70-pioneering-heart-surgeon-is-dead.html. Accessed 15 Dec 209.

25. Carson B, Murphey C. Gifted hands: the Ben Carson story. 20th anniversary ed. Grand Rapids: Zondervan; 2011.

3

Evolution of the Black Physician: Medical Education and Treatment Facilities for Blacks

> ....until that day when a man's color will not lead to his embarrassment....
> until the day when equality of opportunity is incorporated into the actual codes and practices of every American community, we will vitally need our own institutions.
>
> —Black surgeon Frederick Douglass Stubbs, 1944 [1]

> The Negro Hospital in America, like almost all Negro institutions of service and learning, was born in protest to the transitional modes of segregation and discrimination.
>
> —Black surgeon Frederick Douglass Stubbs, 1944 [1]

Introduction

Following the end of the Civil War and the beginning of emancipation (1863–1865), blacks were cast into a situation of having to be responsible for providing their own medical care. Freedom from bondage meant that they could no longer depend on their former slave masters to care for them when they were ill or injured, and they had little or no money to go to white hospitals or physicians, even if they had been accepted for treatment. In the aftermath of a war that was fought to determine the destiny of millions of blacks who were caught in between two factions of whites, there were remarkable efforts to survive.

Precursors of Black Educational and Institutional Development

We begin with the Reconstruction Period which spanned the era from 1865 at the end of the Civil War to 1877. At the beginning of this period, there were virtually no health facilities for the newly freed slaves. Due to the actions of a few influential

© Springer Nature Switzerland AG 2020
R. A. Williams, *Blacks in Medicine*, https://doi.org/10.1007/978-3-030-41960-8_3

people in the US Congress and elsewhere, such as Senator Thaddeus Stevens of Pennsylvania, the Freedmen's Bureau [2] was created to assuage the miserable health circumstances that blacks were suffering. Initiated by an act of Congress in 1865 as the Bureau of Refugees, Freedmen and Abandoned Lands, it was placed under the War Department and had authority over all matters having to do with freedmen and refugees in the former rebel states. They initiated this government agency during what came to be known as the Reconstruction Period, 1865–1877, when the nation was attempting to bind up the wounds of war, as President Lincoln stressed in his Gettysburg Address, and to relieve the agony of slavery. Ex-slaves were promised and were given some limited help with their very survival, although they never received the allegedly promised "forty acres and a mule" for each freed bondsman that was to allow them to make a fresh start on their own. During the Reconstruction Period, the 14th Amendment to the Constitution was passed, ostensibly giving full citizenship rights to the freed slaves. However, there was pushback by Southern antagonists against the perceived new freedoms that ex-slaves were beginning to enjoy, and "Jim Crow" was instituted which was a very repressive practice of discrimination that relegated them to second-class citizenship again, with establishment of separate or segregated facilities for whites and blacks such as hospitals, educational institutions, restaurants, theaters, and transportation in Southern states. More seriously, the infamous Black Codes were instituted, which restricted certain activities by blacks and banned the gathering of more than a small number of blacks in one location at the same time; and the deadly Ku Klux Klan (KKK), the most antiblack group of all, was born in Tennessee.

When the US Supreme Court ruled in favor of the defendant in the case of *Plessy v. Ferguson*, 163 U.S. 537 (1896) [3], the repression of civil rights was confirmed as legal, and it became the basis of the racism that prevails in the United States today, including in medical education and healthcare delivery, although its principles were denounced and repudiated in the US Supreme Court Decision *Brown v. Board of Education of Topeka*, 347 U.S. 483 (1954).

Black Institutions for Medical Education

Between 1865 and 1904, a developmental phenomenon occurred which was to shape the future of black involvement in healthcare in all dimensions for years to come. Motivated by the sheer need to provide their own care and to develop their own physicians and nurses, blacks founded and created medical and nursing institutions which educated a cadre of healthcare professionals to care for themselves. The first of these was Howard University, which was the first land-grant institution of higher learning in the United States. Opened with Federal funding in Washington, D.C. in 1868, Howard had a medical school which was dedicated strictly to the training of black physicians (schools of dentistry, nursing, and pharmacy were added later). Named for Oliver Otis Howard, a white Union general in the Civil War, Howard initially was staffed by white professors and a Caucasian supervisor; eventually, they were replaced by mostly black faculty. Howard also added a clinical element, aptly named Freedmen's Hospital, opened in 1862, which was called one of the finest treatment facilities in the nation. It was headed by Alexander T. Augusta, MD, a former major and surgeon in the US Army. Freedmen's Hospital was originally established to treat former slaves and blacks who served in the Civil War.

Hundreds of black physicians were trained at Howard, which at that time was about the only medical school that openly admitted black students to the study of medicine.

Another black medical school was opened in Nashville, Tennessee, by virtue of an act of sheer human kindness: the Meharry brothers, who were wealthy farmers in that locality, observed the suffering of the black population there after slavery was ended, and they funded the creation of a medical school that was named for them; thus was Meharry Medical College born, in 1876. It actually began as the Meharry Medical Department of Central Tennessee University but later became a full-fledged degree-granting medical school.

In all, 14 black medical schools opened in the nation during this developmental period when blacks were determined to do or die regarding inventing the resources and facilities needed for survival. However, by 1910, all but two of them, Howard and Meharry, were closed, mainly as a consequence of the Flexner Report, which will be described in detail below. The schools that are now defunct, the period during which they operated, and their locations are listed in Table 3.1 [4].

Much of the early medical education prior to the turn of the twentieth century was stimulated by church and religious organizations such as the American Baptist Home Mission Society. In many cases there was no formal medical training; several men became doctors through apprenticeship, which involved attaching oneself to an experienced physician and learning the craft from him. In fact, James Derham or Durham, who is acknowledged to be the first black doctor trained in America, learned medicine from two physicians in Louisiana, and after earning enough to buy his freedom from slavery at age 21, he set up a highly successful practice in New Orleans that led to such envy among white physicians that the city restrained

Table 3.1 Defunct black medical schools in the United States [4]

School/University	City, State	Dates
Lincoln University	Oxford PA	1870–1874
Straight University Medical Department	New Orleans LA	1873–1874
Leonard Medical School, Shaw University	Raleigh NC	1882–1918
Louisville National Medical College	Louisville KY	1888–1912
New Orleans University Medical College (Flint Medical College)	New Orleans LA	1889–1911
Hannibal Medical College	Memphis TN	1889–1896
Knoxville College Medical Department	Knoxville TN	1895–1900
State University Medical Department	Louisville KY	1899–1903
Chattanooga National Medical College	Chattanooga TN	1899–1904
Knoxville Medical College	Knoxville TN	1900–1910
University of West Tennessee College of Physicians and Surgeons	Jackson TN	1900–1907
	Memphis TN	1907–1923
Medico-Chirurgical and Theological College of Christ's Institution	Baltimore MD	1900–1908?

and limited his practice in 1789 ostensibly because of his lack of formal training. This attitude toward practitioners produced by "doctor mills" increased into the early years of the twentieth century, and these commercial medical schools which often admitted students in October and graduated them the following spring came more and more under the scrutiny of the Carnegie Foundation for the Advancement of Teaching, whose president, Henry S. Pritchett, declared that "for 25 years past, there has been an enormous overproduction of uneducated and ill-trained medical practitioners" [5].

Ultimately, the American Medical Association (AMA), the largest medical organization in the United States, took notice of the commercialization of medical education, and it formed the Council on Medical Education in 1904. This assembly joined with the Association of American Medical Colleges (AAMC) and the Carnegie Foundation to decry proprietary schools as menaces which should be regulated, controlled, and in most cases closed down to protect the public. The AMA Council on Medical Education (ACME) set standards for reforming medical schools which involved standardizing admission requirements and establishing curriculum standards requiring basic science and laboratory study followed by clinical experience in teaching hospitals. However, it was necessary for a thorough investigation of medical schools throughout the country to be conducted to determine which schools needed special attention. The thrust for this effort was provided by the Carnegie Foundation, which commissioned a non-physician, Dr. Abraham Flexner, to take on this ambitious project (Fig. 3.1).

Over an 18-month period, Dr. Flexner visited 155 medical schools and issued his report in 1910. It was apocalyptic for several institutions, and particularly for the seven black schools that were still functioning up to that time. These included Shaw University-Leonard Medical School, Raleigh, NC, est. 1882; Flint Medical College of New Orleans University, est. 1873; Hannibal Medical College, Memphis, TN, est.1889; Chattanooga National Medical College, Chattanooga, TN, est. 1899; Louisville National Medical College, Louisville, KY, est. 1888; and the University of West Tennessee College of Physicians and Surgeons, Jackson, TN, est. 1900. Flexner's pronouncements led to the closing of all but two of the black schools, Howard and Meharry, which he found meritorious enough to remain open with some recommended changes to be made. For instance, Flexner stated that these two black schools should concentrate on producing "sanitarians" (instead of surgeons), whose role should be to create a non-infectious environment among black patients for the protection of whites by controlling this "source of contagion" ("Ten million of them live in close contact with sixty million whites....The Negro must be educated not only for his sake, but for ours....") [6]. His book, *Medical Education in the United States and Canada: A Report to the Carnegie Foundation for the Advancement of Teaching and Education*, created instant changes on the medical school scene that reverberate to this day [6]. Hundreds of black physicians had been produced by the black medical schools prior to the Flexner Report, and there was a rapid decline in the production of new black physicians which still persists. The continued lack of education of blacks to become physicians is one of the key contributors to the "slave health deficit" described by Byrd and Clayton in their monumental book, *An*

Fig. 3.1 Abraham Flexner, MD. (From Hollinger WM. The world's work, Vol XX May to Oct 1910. A history of our time. Garden City NY: Doubleday, Page & Co. 1910. https://archive.org/stream/worldswork 20gard#page/13100/mode/2up, Public Domain, https://commons.wikimedia.org/w/index.php?curid=26650987)

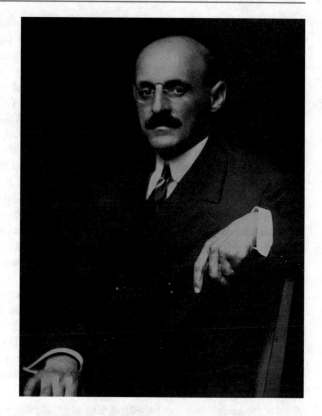

American Health Dilemma [7]. This deficiency still persists despite the opening of two more schools dedicated to producing and educating black physicians in addition to Howard and Meharry: Charles R. Drew University of Medicine and Science, Los Angeles, CA, est. 1966, and Morehouse School of Medicine, Atlanta, GA, est. 1975. More information and history of this period can be obtained from an excellent 2006 paper by Harley [4].

Black-Owned and Black-Operated Hospitals

Similar to what was stated above about the need that blacks had for medical educational facilities of their own in order to produce their own physicians, there was a parallel need for facilities including hospitals and clinics to treat them. Although many white hospitals did not admit or treat black patients at all, some of them did admit blacks on a limited basis but relegated them to segregated black wards away from white patients. These "colored wards" were often in the basement or some other isolated location. Black physicians were not allowed to practice in these hospitals, not even on their own patients [8].

In 1832, the first black hospital was founded in Savannah, GA, and by 1928, spurred by segregation, there were about 183 facilities that could be identified as black-owned and black-operated hospitals. Hospital limitations on black medical school graduates meant that only a few were open for internships and residencies for training in a few fields such as family practice, obstetrics and gynecology, midwifery, and pediatrics, according to Watson [9]. Some of the teaching hospitals that were owned and operated by blacks and that accepted black physicians for postgraduate training were Freedmen's Hospital, associated with Howard University School of Medicine in Washington, DC (1866 to the present and currently Howard University Hospital); Provident Hospital of Chicago (1891–1988); Provident Hospital of Baltimore, MD (1894–1986); Flint-Goodridge Hospital, New Orleans, LA (1901–1985); Frederick Douglass Hospital and Training School of Philadelphia (Fig. 3.2), founded in 1895, which later became Mercy-Douglass Hospital and closed in 1973; Hubbard Hospital, Nashville, TN, which was associated with Meharry Medical School, 1910–1994; Homer G. Phillips Hospital, St. Louis, MO (1937–recent); and the Tuskegee Veterans Administration Medical Center (1923–present).

Surgical training was essentially off-limits to blacks until breakthroughs by a small number of physicians in the last half of the nineteenth century [10]. However, that number fell to less than 80 by 1965. Thus, there was a rise and fall, as Wesley describes it, of black hospitals between 1832 and 1965 [11]. This phenomenon was undoubtedly influenced by national politics such as the passage of the Hill-Burton Hospital Survey and Construction Act. It is important to understand the impact that

Fig. 3.2 Frederick Douglass Memorial Hospital and Training School, c. 1910. Goin' North, accessed January 4, 2020, https://goinnorth.org/items/show/988. (Courtesy The African American Museum in Philadelphia)

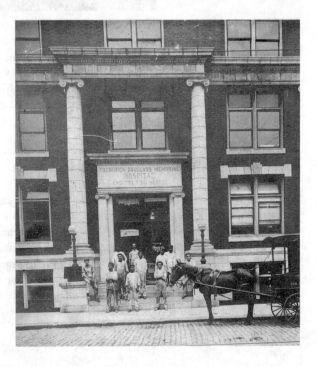

this legislation had on the fate and destiny of black health professionals and black patients during this critical period of the development of black medicine. We will now analyze it in some detail.

Between 1929, when the American stock market crashed and the country was plunged into the Great Depression, and 1945, when World War II ended, public accommodations such as hospitals, clinics, and nursing homes fell into a state of disrepair and dysfunction due to the deployment of resources and funds to the war effort and more immediate needs. Within 2 months after the war ended, President Harry S. Truman spoke to the nation about a five-point plan to restore many essential public services and to rebuild the nation's healthcare delivery infrastructure. In a special message to Congress, he outlined a bold program designed to restore the integrity of American healthcare. The first of his proposals called for the construction of hospitals and related health facilities, and it became the basis for the Hospital Survey and Construction Act, better known as the Hill-Burton Act in recognition of its sponsors, Republican Senator Harold Burton of Ohio and Senator Lister Hill, a Democrat from Alabama [12]. It was passed by Congress as a bipartisan initiative that had three principal aims: to refurbish existing healthcare facilities and to modernize them; to construct new healthcare resources to serve a growing American population which was also being increased by the hundreds of thousands of those returning from military duty; and to provide the South, which suffered more from insufficient medical facilities than other parts of the United States, with a much-needed stimulus (40% of the nation's counties had no hospitals at all in 1945; most of these counties without hospitals were in the South). President Truman signed Hill-Burton into law on August 13, 1946. It provided $3.7 billion in Federal funding and $9.1 billion in matching grants from state and local governments. As such, it was the first large-scale involvement of the Federal Government in funding healthcare and was in a real sense the predecessor of the Affordable Care Act of today. The South benefited more than any other part of the country, with half of the new hospitals being built there. Over the years since its initiation to 1971, Hill-Burton was responsible for the construction of almost 500,000 hospital beds in 10,748 projects around the country [12]. By 1975, nearly one-third of new hospitals were built with Hill-Burton funds. One of those hospitals was the Moses H. Cone Memorial Hospital in Greensboro, NC (Fig. 3.3), which was the focus of a monumental desegregation court case in 1963, described below. By the turn of the twenty-first century, 6800 facilities in 4000 communities had been funded by Hill-Burton, so it came to be an enormously impactful measure which accrued to the public benefit.

However, although the Hill-Burton Act was certainly beneficial in bolstering a failing healthcare system in the last half of the twentieth century, it had some glitches that needed correction. Although the initial legislation required that facilities receiving Hill-Burton funding were not allowed to discriminate based on race, color, national origin, or creed, a curious compromise was reached with white hospitals that still wanted to exclude black patients and physicians while accepting the government money. A general agreement was entered into through a clause in the bill that allowed separation of whites and blacks so long as the facilities, wards, clinics, etc. were equal. Thus, segregation continued in white healthcare facilities;

Fig. 3.3 Construction of the Moses H. Cone Memorial Hospital in Greensboro, NC, was partially funded by the Hill-Burton Act. The hospital, seen circa 1973, was at the center of a court case that brought an end to racially segregated healthcare. (Courtesy Cone Health Medical Library, with permission)

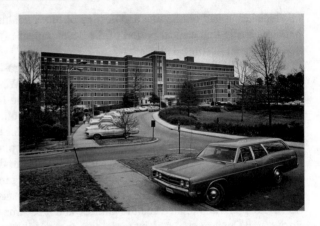

although it was prohibited by law, segregation was codified by that very law by virtue of the *separate but equal* clause. This clause emanated from a Supreme Court decision in 1896; in *Plessy v. Ferguson*, the Court held that states could impose segregation as long as they provided similar facilities to blacks and whites. Thus, the vast majority of Southern hospitals still discriminated against blacks while reaping the benefits of Hill-Burton funding.

Separate but equal was supported by some pundits who felt that it provided at least some improvement in the dire healthcare discrimination picture confronting blacks, because a few more of them were able to take advantage of the new Hill-Burton facilities. Edward H. Beardsley, whose excellent book about healthcare in the South, *A History of Neglect: Health Care for Blacks and Mill Workers in the Twentieth Century South*, which I reviewed for the *Journal of the American Medical Association* in 1987, was among those who felt that blacks derived some advantages from separate but equal by gaining a small amount of access where there was none before [13]. However, the eminent civil rights activist, NAACP president (1976–1982), brilliant scholar, historian, and Howard University medical professor, Dr. W. Montague Cobb (Fig. 3.4) once related to me that he did not view separate but equal as an improvement; as he stated, "the government can hardly handle one deficient medical system. How in the world will they be able to manage two?" Calling the old system "Jim Crow" and the new Hill-Burton system "deluxe Jim Crow" [14], he launched a torrid legal and political crusade against hospital segregation and discrimination in general which carried on for years. During these battles, he visited with presidents at the White House and traveled widely throughout the South to encourage black physicians and citizens to sue hospitals and local governments for equal treatment. The Imhotep Conferences which he instituted were a series of meetings at the White House designed to create a dialogue on two key issues: racial discrimination in medical education, and hospital segregation. The meetings were held annually from 1957 to 1964, concluding when the Civil Rights Act was signed, which was heavily influenced by these encounters.

This nefarious aversion of equity in healthcare delivery persisted until 1963 when Dr. Hubert Eaton, a black physician in Greensboro, NC, brought suit against

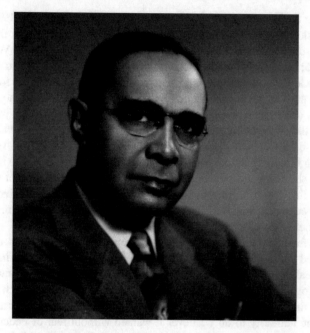

Fig. 3.4 W. Montague Cobb, MD, PhD (1904–1990), the quintessential historian of African Americans in Medicine. A graduate of Amherst and Howard University College of Medicine, he also received a PhD degree in Anatomy and Anthropology and subsequently served as Chair of the Department of Anatomy at Howard. He was an ardent civil rights activist whose lobbying efforts with presidents at the White House helped in the passage of the Civil Rights Act of 1964 and of Medicare in 1965. Dr. Cobb was also president of the NAACP and of the National Medical Association. (Courtesy National Library of Medicine Digital Collection. NLM Unique ID: 101412157; with kind permission from the Cobb family)

a hospital that had denied privileges to him for admitting and treating his patients. The lawsuit, *Simkins v. Moses H. Cone Memorial Hospital*, was a blockbuster case that finally brought an end to segregated healthcare [15]. Technically, the *Simkins v. Cone* case was decided in favor of the plaintiffs, including Dr. Eaton, when the US Supreme Court denied *certiorari* to the 4th Circuit Court of Appeals decision. Another important provision of the decision was that free care for poor people, including impoverished black citizens, was required of hospitals receiving Federal funds. Thus, a statute that was originally intended to bring equity of opportunity into the American healthcare delivery scene, but then was perverted by those of racist persuasion, was eventually returned to the path of righteousness by brave pioneers like Dr. Hubert Eaton, whose unselfish determination to achieve justice would not be denied. He is a true hero of the struggle against segregation and racial discrimination.

The period encompassing 1939 through 1965 was a critical span of time for progress in healthcare for blacks, especially in the South. During this period, a number of important pieces of legislation were passed which impacted upon discrimination in public accommodations. These included the initiation of a national health plan in

1939 during the Roosevelt administration; Hill-Burton in 1947; the 1954 Supreme Court decision in *Brown v. Board of Education of Topeka*, Kansas that declared segregated schools unconstitutional; the Civil Rights Act of 1964; the Voting Rights Act of 1965; and passage of legislation creating Medicare and Medicaid in 1965. All of these legislative changes represented seismic upheavals in the foundation of society and particularly in healthcare for our citizens, and it must be noted that they were in part driven by civil rights activism which occurred in parallel with the legal precedents that were being established. This included vigorous activism and support for these measures by the National Medical Association (NMA). As Dr. Martin Luther King famously stated, "of all the forms of inequality, injustice in healthcare is the most shocking and inhumane" (Second National Convention of the Medical Committee for Human Rights, Chicago, 1966), and correcting these inequities was at the very center of the civil rights program, including integrating medical treatment facilities (Fig. 3.5).

Federal financing of hospitals and government funding of new construction largely faded out in 1997, but not before establishing a Federal footprint in the provision of healthcare for those unable to afford it. The effect of this new thrust created a controversy over government involvement in public affairs which resonates to the present time. Questions arose about states' rights, that is, whether an individual state had the authority to do whatever it wanted without fear of Federal intervention, regulation, or, as some might say, interference. Originally, this issue had been visited after the Civil War, when there was intense debate in Congress over the right of states to declare whether former slaves were citizens with all rights that should accrue to such persons. Although slavery itself had been abolished by the Thirteenth Amendment to the Constitution which had been ratified on December 6, 1865 following intense debate in Congress and support from President Abraham Lincoln, the rights of those freed men were not clearly established, especially regarding such freedoms as voting in elections. Even though another statute, the Civil Rights Act of 1866, was enacted, their status was still not clearly defined.

This created the rationale for the Fourteenth Amendment to the US Constitution, whose major provision was to grant and to guarantee equal legal and civil rights to

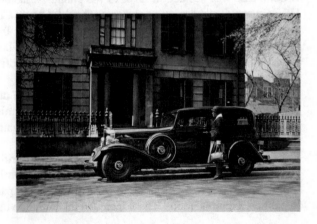

Fig. 3.5 Savannah Health Center (1894–1953), a facility that was limited to the treatment of blacks. A black nurse is standing by an automobile that is used to transport nurses to the districts under their care. (Courtesy National Library of Medicine Digital Collection. NLM Unique ID: 101441642)

"All persons born or naturalized in the United States." It thereby granted citizenship to former slaves which was backed up by the Constitution. It was ratified on July 28, 1868, including a declaration that "nor shall any state deprive any person of life, liberty, or property, without due process of law, nor deny to any person within its jurisdiction equal protection of the laws." It was supposed to extend liberties and rights granted by the Bill of Rights to the former slaves.

Importantly, the Citizenship Clause of the Fourteenth Amendment overruled the Dred Scott decision of 1857, which had ruled that black people were not and could not be citizens because a black man represented only three-fifths of a white man and therefore "had no rights that a white man was bound to respect" [16]. Thus, the Fourteenth Amendment should be viewed as the document that provided the greatest measure of freedom for blacks at that time, more so than the Emancipation Proclamation or the Thirteenth Amendment.

Conclusion

It must be recognized, based on these legal events that occurred from the middle of the nineteenth century to the present, that the pathway to freedom which blacks had to walk was not an easy, straightforward road, and in fact it was often tortuous, dangerous, and deadly. Even when the US government declared that blacks had been given "inalienable rights" as bona fide citizens of the United States, those freedoms were often retracted in actual life, and these challenges still occur on the healthcare scene with the denial of true equity. This persistent lack of equity has its most harmful effect in the healthcare arena, where it translates into higher morbidity and mortality rates for blacks. This is where the clinical impact is seen on the health and lives of blacks in America. This demonstrates the interaction and connectivity between race, ethnicity, politics, socioeconomics, and racism, with healthcare disparities resulting from this toxic mixture. We should give special credit to Wilbur H. Watson for pointing this out to us in his groundbreaking book, *Against the Odds* [9].

References

1. Stubbs FD. The purpose of the community hospital. Nat Med Assoc. 1944;3(5):152–4.
2. Colby IC. The Freedmen's Bureau: from social welfare to segregation. Phylon (1960-). 1985;46(3):219–30.
3. Fireside H. Separate and unequal: Homer Plessy and the Supreme Court decision that legalized racism. New York: Caroll & Graf; 2004.
4. Harley EH. The forgotten history of defunct black medical schools in the 19th and 20th centuries and the impact of the Flexner report. J Nat Med Assoc. 2006;98(9):1425–9.
5. Savitt TL. Abraham Flexner and the black medical schools. In: Baransky BM, Gevitz N, editors. Beyond Flexner: medical education in the twentieth century. Contributions in medical studies, Number 34. Westport: Greenwood Press; 1992.
6. Flexner A. Medical education in the United States and Canada: a report to the Carnegie Foundation for the Advancement of Teaching. New York: Bulletin (Carnegie Foundation) No. 4; 1910.

7. Byrd WM, Clayton LA. An American health dilemma: a medical history of African Americans and the problem of race: beginnings to 1900, vol. 1. New York/London: Routledge; 2000.
8. Hine DC. Health and the Afro-American family. In: Health. Washington, DC: Associated Publishers; 1984. p. 2.
9. Watson WH. Against the odds: blacks in the profession of medicine in the United States. Abingdon/New York: Transaction Publishers/Routledge/Taylor & Francis; 1999.
10. Organ CH Jr, Kosiba MM. A century of black surgeons: the U.S.A. experience. Norman: Transcript Press; 1987.
11. Wesley NM. Searching for survival: black hospitals listing and selected commentary: searching for survival. Washington, DC: Health Services Administration Dept., School of Business and Public Administration, Howard University; 1983.
12. Thomas KK. The Hill-Burton Act and civil rights: expanding hospital care for black southerners, 1939-1960. J South Hist. 2006;72(4):823–70.
13. Beardsley EH. A history of neglect. Health care for blacks and mill workers in the twentieth-century south. Knoxville: University of Tennessee Press; 1987.
14. Cobb WM. The crushing irony of deluxe Jim Crow (editorial). J Nat Med Assoc. 1952;44(5):386–7.
15. Reynolds PP. Hospitals and civil rights, 1945-1963: the case of Simkins v Moses H. Cone Memorial Hospital. Ann Intern Med. 1997;126(11):898–906.
16. Maltz EM. Dred Scott and the politics of slavery. (Landmark Law Cases & American Society) Lawrence: University Press of Kansas. p. 115.

The Impact of Black Medical Organizations on African American Health

4

A legendary late poet spoke to the horrible conditions:
>Out of the huts of history's shame
>I rise
>Up from a past that's rooted in pain
>I rise
>I'm a black ocean, leaping and wide,
>Welling and swelling I bear in the tide.
>Leaving behind nights of terror and fear
>I rise
>Into a daybreak that's wondrously clear
>I rise
>Bringing the gifts that my ancestors gave,
>I am the dream and the hope of the slave.
>I rise
>I rise
>I rise.
>– Maya Angelou

Introduction

The previous chapters have explored the impact that individuals, ideas, and institutions have had on black lives in America. We have given an account of the black physicians who were medical pioneers in the black community, including the early slave doctors and the first licensed African American medical pioneers who came upon the scene in the nineteenth and early twentieth centuries. We also considered some of the medical ideology, such as folk medicine, that affected the black population, and we presented the evidence that blacks in this country have been subjected to a long tradition of discrimination and racial segregation that has resulted in inferior and substandard healthcare delivery for this segment of the population. We looked deeply into the educational evolution of black physicians and examined the development of medical schools that focused on teaching them as well as hospitals that provided postgraduate training for them.

© Springer Nature Switzerland AG 2020
R. A. Williams, *Blacks in Medicine*, https://doi.org/10.1007/978-3-030-41960-8_4

This chapter will continue the story of how black people took charge of their own healthcare and how they established a well-defined footprint in the annals of medicine. It deals with a presentation of the two major black medical organizations impacting black healthcare whose development spanned the period from the late nineteenth century to the present time. No realistic and meaningful discussion about healthcare for African Americans can be carried on without including these two giants in the conversation. I am able to write knowledgably about both, because I am privileged to have been at one time the president of the first organization, the National Medical Association (NMA), and the founder and former president of the second, the Association of Black Cardiologists (ABC). I present a historical and expository presentation on each one and will provide an analysis of the impact that each has had on blacks in medicine over the past 120-plus years.

The History of the National Medical Association

The National Medical Association (NMA) was founded in 1895 by 12 black physicians attending the Cotton States and International Exposition in Atlanta, Georgia, where Booker T. Washington delivered his historic "Atlanta Compromise speech" [1] in which he articulated the (submissive) role that Negroes should play in American society in order to coexist with whites:

> In all things that are purely social, we can be as separate as the fingers, yet one as the hand in all things essential to mutual progress.… The wisest among my race understand that the agitation of questions of social equality is the extremist folly, and that progress in the enjoyment of all the privileges that will come to us must be the result of severe and constant struggle rather than of artificial forcing.

The physicians met at the First Congregational Church in Atlanta (Fig. 4.1) [2] and decided to start a medical organization of their own after being continually rebuffed and refused admission by the American Medical Association (AMA), which was established in 1847. At first they called their new organization the National Association of Colored Physicians, Dentists, and Pharmacists but later changed the name to the current NMA.

The NMA's historical credo, written by one of the founding fathers, C.V. Roman, MD, poetically demonstrates what frustrations lay beneath the beginning of the organization but also shows the purpose and the intensity of the founders' resolve to create a venerable group that African American physicians could call "home." The NMA credo was articulated by Dr. Roman in his response to the welcome addresses at the NMA's annual meeting in New York City in August 1908 [3]:

> Conceived in no spirit of racial exclusiveness, fostering no ethnic antagonism, but born of the exigencies of the American environment, the National Medical Association has for its object the banding together for mutual cooperation and helpfulness, the men and women of African descent who are legally and honorably engaged in the practice of the cognate professions of medicine, surgery, pharmacy and dentistry.

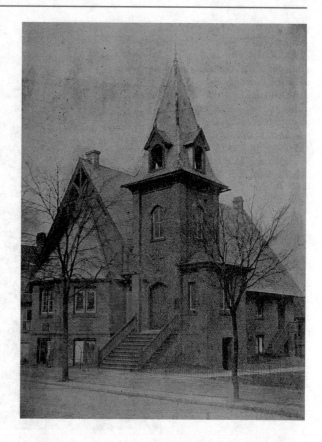

Fig. 4.1 The First
Congregational Church,
Atlanta: Site of the
meeting that founded.
(From Penn and Bowen
[2]; scanned from original
in Library of Wellesley
College https://commons.
wikimedia.org/wiki/
File:The_united_negro-_
his_problems_and_his_
progress,_containing_the_
addresses_and_
proceedings_the_Negro_
young_people%27s_
Christian_and_
educational_congress,_
held_August_6-11,_1902;_
(1902)_
(14761746596).jpg)

Dr. Robert F. Boyd of Nashville, TN, served as the first president of the NMA (see Chap. 6), and Dr. Daniel Hale Williams of Chicago, IL, became the vice president. Others in this founding group included Dr. Miles Vanderhurst Lynk of Memphis, TN; Daniel L. Martin, MD of Nashville, TN, secretary; David H.C. Scott, MD of Montgomery, AL, treasurer; and H.R. Butler, MD of Atlanta, GA, chairman of the executive committee. Dr. Daniel Hale Williams (Fig. 4.2) had achieved fame by performing the first operation of any kind on the human heart at Provident Hospital in Chicago in 1893 [4]; and as mentioned above, Dr. C.V. Roman, who became the first editor of the *Journal of the National Medical Association* in 1908 (Fig. 4.3) [5], was also a charter member of the NMA. They began their mission to "advance the art and science of medicine for people of African descent" through education, advocacy, and health policy. Figure 4.4 is a historical photograph showing the NMA members gathered at a convention in Boston in 1909.

Almost from the beginning of its existence, the NMA joined in the debate on national health insurance that was initiated by US President Theodore Roosevelt in the early years of the twentieth century. There was vigorous discussion of President Roosevelt's revolutionary plan to provide healthcare insurance coverage for all

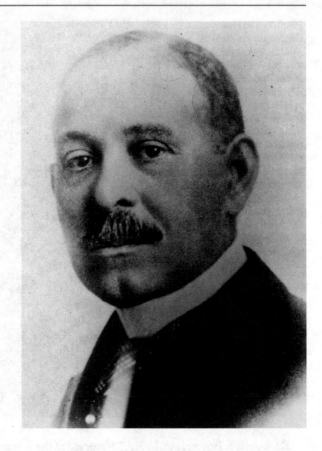

Fig. 4.2 Daniel Hale Williams, MD (1856–1931), Founding member of the National Medical Association. In 1893, he performed the first operation on the living human heart. (Courtesy National Library of Medicine Digital Collection. NLM Unique ID:101448033)

Americans [6], a position that the NMA strongly supported because it promised to guarantee healthcare for the black population as well as for the rest of the nation. By 1910, the debate raged across the country and into the halls of Congress where it was defeated following opposition by the AMA. Thus, the first (unsuccessful) attempt to enact healthcare reform on a national basis occurred in 1910, 100 years before the Affordable Care Act was written into law by President Barack Obama on March 23, 2010. However, the larger story here is that the NMA became the champion of equity in healthcare delivery, in contrast to the AMA, which opposed comprehensive health insurance.

The NMA was incorporated in 1924. In 2020, it will observe its 125th year of continuous operation. During all of that time, a complete history of the NMA has never been written.

As time passed, the NMA grew into a sizable organization, representing the interests of 40,000 mostly black medical practitioners and African American patients. As such, it has become the largest and oldest black medical organization in the world, with more than 112 affiliates and societies in the United States and its territories. With administrative headquarters in Silver Spring, MD, it consists of 25 specialty sections ranging from aerospace medicine to women's health. Governed by a Board of Trustees

Fig. 4.3 The Editors of the Journal of the National Medical Association, 1914. Charles V. Roman, MD, is seated in the center. From left to right: John A. Kenney, Sr., MD; Walter A. Alexander, MD; Roscoe C. Brown, MD; and Ulysses G. Dailey, MD. (Courtesy History of Medicine Division, National Library of Medicine) [5]

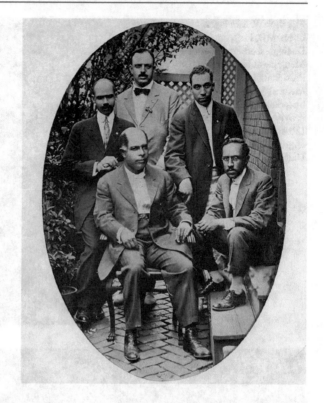

operating under its constitution and bylaws as a 501C3 nonprofit corporation, it carries out numerous programs led by an executive director; it is designed to benefit the public interest and to address the special needs of the black population. Its most comprehensive areas of focus are on eliminating healthcare disparities, achieving social justice, increasing diversity in the medical field, and promoting healthcare reform.

It must be acknowledged, for historical accuracy, that the NMA was actually preceded by another organization as the first black medical society, as pointed out by the brilliant historian, Dr. W. Montague Cobb [7] (Fig. 4.5). Officially formed in Washington, DC, on April 21, 1884, in the office of Dean Robert Reyburn, MD of Howard University School of Medicine, and called The Medico-Chirurgical Society of the District of Columbia ("Med-Chi"), its creation was chronicled in a small book entitled *The First Negro Medical Society* written by Dr. Cobb in 1939 [8]. The creation of Med-Chi was actually set in motion in 1869 when three black physicians in Washington, DC, A. T. Augusta, C.B. Purvis, and A.W. Tucker, applied for admission to the Medical Society of the District of Columbia (MSDC), an all-white group of practitioners that was approved by Congress to be the official medical organization in Washington, a federal district. As such, they were required by their government charter to accept all medically qualified individuals who applied for membership regardless of race or ethnicity. However, notwithstanding this dictum, all three black applicants were rejected by vote of the MSDC membership, and

Fig. 4.4 W. Montague Cobb, MD, PhD, Distinguished Professor of Medicine at Howard, Past President of the National Medical Association, historian, and Civil Rights activist. (Courtesy National Library of Medicine Digital Collection. NLM Unique ID: 101412157)

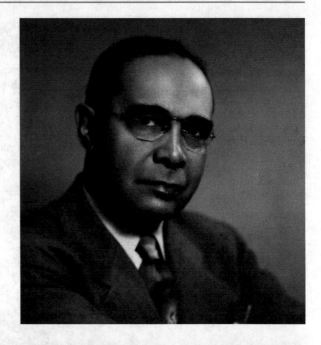

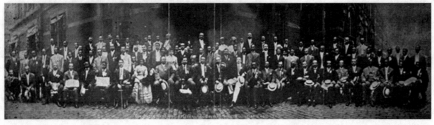

Fig. 4.5 The National Medical Association–National Convention, Boston, Massachusetts, August 24–26, 1909. (Courtesy National Library of Medicine https://www.nlm.nih.gov/exhibition/afram-surgeons/history.html)

they were also subsequently rebuffed when they formed a new group called the National Medical Society (NMS) in 1870 and went onto the floor of Congress in an effort to have MSDC's charter repealed. This endeavor also failed despite the heroic efforts of the eminent civil rights activist Senator Charles Sumner of Massachusetts (Fig. 4.6), who sponsored an amendment to the first Civil Rights Act of 1866 in an attempt to increase amenities for blacks in travel, public accommodations, education, and healthcare. They were also denied admission to the AMA by virtue of having been rejected by the local medical society. As a consequence, they decided to establish Med-Chi.

The exclusive policies of MSDC and its affiliates continued for 83 years until they were finally reversed in 1952. By that time, the NMA had been formed, and Med-Chi became an affiliate organization. It was already 11 years old by the time that the NMA was founded in 1895. Med-Chi has played an important role in black

Fig. 4.6 Senator Charles Sumner, civil rights and anti-slavery activist who was nearly beaten to death in 1856 by a fellow senator on the floor of the US Congress for expressing his views. (Original daguerreotype in Rare Books Department, Boston Public Library: BPLDC: Date: 1855) (approximate) (By unknown, scanned by BPL – Charles Sumner Uploaded by Trycatch, CC BY 2.0, https://commons.wikimedia.org/w/index.php?curid=9687494)

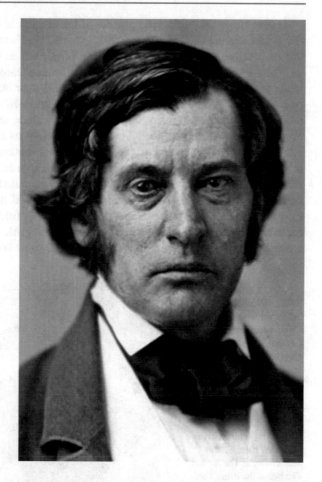

medical history, including challenging the tradition carried on by whites of excluding blacks from practicing in local hospitals in the District of Columbia. One successful example was their effort to open Gallinger Municipal Hospital, later known as DC General Hospital, to black practitioners in 1948. Med-Chi also is credited with initiating the Imhotep National Conference on Hospital Integration, which was held each year at the White House with presidential sponsorship from 1957 to 1964 and was largely presided over by Dr. Cobb, a prominent member of Med-Chi.

The emergence of the NMA despite severe obstacles placed in the paths of black physicians is a phenomenon unequalled in the annals of medicine. The situation is summed up in excellent fashion by Dr. M.V. Lynk [9]:

> Coming out of a background of slavery and almost complete illiteracy, hampered in his efforts to get even elementary education and, then, once this obstacle was leveled and the educational requisites secured, frustrated and stymied by the closed door policies of the established medical colleges and hospitals, the negro doctor has had to struggle in a fashion and with a persistency rarely, if ever, equaled by any other group seeking professional status.

One of the most unfortunate aspects of the attempt to establish collegial inter-racial relations between blacks and whites in medicine is that instead of welcoming and embracing the new African American physicians as colleagues and embracing them as brothers in a joint effort to uplift healthcare for all, the mainstream white medical profession rejected and suppressed their emergence, evolution, and education [10]. While it is impossible to determine why there has been so much resistance on the part of many whites in medical circles, societies, institutions, and organizations to accept African American physicians as colleagues, brothers, and sisters in medical practice, hospitals, and medical schools, it is easy to speculate based on several lines of evidence that this resistance is caused by pure unadulterated racism. For example, there is an expression called "colorphobia" that was used to explain why the white gentleman physicians of the MSDC and the AMA refused to accept and admit black physicians into their folds. Figure 4.7 is an actual expression of how many whites have historically regarded blacks in general from a physical or physiological standpoint and is the spirit behind the Jim Crow laws

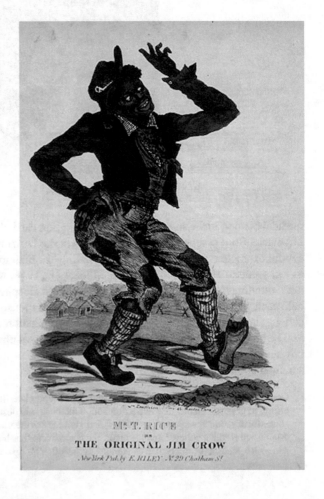

Fig. 4.7 Cartoon by Edward Williams Clay of the mythical character Jim Crow, which mocked black physical and physiological characteristics. It became the symbol of racist practices in the United States. (Cover to an early edition of *Jump Jim Crow* sheet music. Thomas D. Rice is pictured in his blackface role; he was performing at The Bowery Theatre at the time. This image was highly influential on later Jim Crow and minstrelsy images. From original in Institute for Advanced Technology in the Humanities at the University of Virginia: Home – pic. Public Domain, https://commons.wikimedia.org/w/index.php?curid=391950)

enacted after 1865 that prevented social interactions between blacks and whites and prevented significant advancements by African Americans. Figure 4.8 is a cartoonist's depiction of the blunt perception that was held by many white physicians about black physicians who were interested in joining their ranks. Such uncomplimentary thinking and the lampooning of black physicians' efforts to become medically self-sufficient represents the mendacity of racism at its ugliest. It is amazing that blacks did not revolt against the white medical establishment for the maltreatment, rejection, and discrimination that they suffered; instead, to their credit, they opted to take the high road and to create their own destiny. The NMA is the direct result of their determination to be autonomous, relevant, potent, and effective in providing lifesaving care for their people.

The NMA deserves credit for rescuing the black physician from the grip of prejudice and denial of his right to pursue a productive practice of medicine, and for fighting for his right to be included in the mainstream of American healthcare provision. It has also fought for the rights of black citizens and others to receive the highest standard of healthcare delivery by successfully battling for the passage of Social Security, Medicare, and Medicaid when the AMA was opposed to these entitlement programs. The group lobbied Congress in support of the Voting Rights Act of 1964

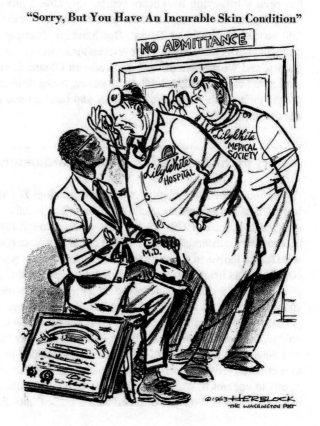

Fig. 4.8 "Sorry, but you have an incurable skin condition" editorial cartoon (by Herbert Block published in *The Washington Post* 4 Jul 1963) depicting white physicians' attitudes toward fraternizing with black physicians as colleagues in white medical societies. (©1963 by Herblock, *The Washington Post.* With permission of the Herb Block Foundation, Washington, DC)

"Sorry, But You Have An Incurable Skin Condition"

NO ADMITTANCE

Lily White HOSPITAL

Lily White MEDICAL SOCIETY

M.D.

©1963 HERBLOCK
THE WASHINGTON POST

and helped Dr. Martin Luther King, Jr., to bring pressure on the government to pass the Civil Rights Act in 1965. It supported *Roe v. Wade* in 1973 in the battle over a woman's right to abortion, and it has been a backer of government backing of Planned Parenthood. (The AMA, on the other hand, was staunchly opposed to abortion, and in 1859 it urged that women who underwent abortion be criminalized, a stand that remained the organization's official policy until 1967, and a stand that has been repeated by the Trump administration.)

In 1973, I was invited to represent the NMA on the iconic American news and talk morning television program *The Today Show* that airs on NBC. I was questioned as to why the NMA was needed since America already had the AMA, a question suggesting perhaps at duplication of effort, and thus a waste of money and resources. I briefly explained that, although both organizations shared a desire to improve healthcare delivery for the entire population, the NMA had the additional obligation of representing the *special* medical and societal needs of African Americans that the AMA had traditionally overlooked. In other words, I attempted to articulate the theme that "black lives matter" in the medical context some decades before the concept was championed by civil rights advocates and protesters.

The NMA also strongly supported the passage of the Patient Protection and Affordable Care Act in 2010 [11], better known as the ACA or Obamacare, which has been a lifesaving healthcare reform measure. Unfortunately, this measure is being threatened with repeal at the present time under the new federal administration headed by President Trump. But however daunting this turn of events may seem, the NMA has a history of overcoming adversity during its long and turbulent history, and we are determined, as President Obama advised shortly after he was elected to his first term in 2008, to be among those Americans who were not afraid to "put their hands on the arc of history and bend it once more toward the hope of a better day" [12].

History of the Association of Black Cardiologists

As the founder of Association of Black Cardiologists (ABC), I can verify that it was born of the exigencies of the unfit American healthcare system as I witnessed it in the 1960s and 1970s while I was going through my medical training. I had become very concerned about the dire conditions under which African Americans were forced to live, in poverty and destitution, and I was particularly concerned about how little was being done to change these circumstances. As I researched the situation around the country, I observed an aura of hopelessness in black communities and a lack of encouragement of black youth to rise above their surroundings and to pursue any meaningful careers such as in what we now call STEM (science, technology, engineering, and math) that might lead to a way out of their constraints and into fields such as healthcare. This attitude that resided in the black community led to a culture of despair that was responsible in part for spawning some grassroots efforts to counter it, such as the wave of civil rights activism that reached its peak during the 1960s. This wave turned into a tide of anti-discrimination and a flood of protests against bigotry and the lack of recognition of the needs and rights of blacks in all areas including healthcare. The Black Power movement, which was an earlier version of the current Black Lives Matter campaign, was born during that time, and the protests boiled over into a turbulent expression of the frustration and anguish that culminated in civil disobedience against repressive white authoritarianism. Ultimately, as these expressions grew, riots, which many prefer to call uprisings, insurrections, or rebellions, began to occur. This was also the time when a number of black civil rights organizations had their beginnings or were strengthened, including the Black Muslims; the Black Panthers; the Southern Christian Leadership Conference (SCLC), established in 1957 by Rev. Dr. Martin Luther King, Jr.; the National Urban League, led by Whitney Young; and the National Association for the Advancement of Colored People (NAACP), co-founded by W.E.B. DuBois in 1909 and later led by Walter White and Roy Wilkins.

One of the most ground-shaking giant civil disturbances was the Watts riots, sometimes referred to as the Watts Rebellion, which raged from August 11 to 16, 1965, in the mostly black South Central region of Los Angeles, where I lived at the time. It began as a protest against police brutality, when a young black motorist, Marquette Frye, was pulled over and arrested by a white California Highway Patrol motorcycle officer, for suspicion of driving while intoxicated. As a crowd of onlookers gathered at the scene of Frye's arrest, strained tensions between police officers and the crowd erupted in a violent exchange. Word spread of his arrest, and shortly afterward, the riot broke out, and chaos ensued. Police and military forces descended on the rioters and turned the city into a battlefield, resulting in more than 40 million dollars' worth of property damage; 34 people were killed in what has been called the worst race riot in US history, which also resulted in more than 1000 reported injuries and almost 4000 arrests before order was restored on August 17.

In the months that followed, many investigations were conducted in an attempt to determine the cause of the riot. In 1965 the State of California convened the McCone Commission, headed by former Central Intelligence Agency head John McCone, and in 1967 the federal government established the National Advisory Commission on Civil Disorders, better known as the Kerner Commission, headed by former Ohio Governor Otto Kerner, to look into this disturbance. The reports of both groups indicated that the root causes included racial disparities in several areas, including education, employment, housing, and healthcare delivery. Both groups also had similar recommendations for fixing the problems such as improved relations between police and the black community, provision of more affordable housing, more job-training programs, improved education, better public transportation, and improvement of healthcare delivery [13].

Not long after the Watts Rebellion, on May 7, 1966, a black man was shot dead when he refused to stop his car while he was rushing his pregnant wife across miles of that vast city from where he lived in the Watts ghetto to the Los Angeles County/ USC Medical Center, where he was taking her to have their baby delivered. The McCone Commission specifically pointed out that a hospital was needed in South Central Los Angeles to care for the medical needs of the poor blacks and other minorities in that location, which would address the situation of health deprivation that necessitated that fatal trip of a desperate husband to get medical attention for his pregnant wife [14]. Interestingly, this became known as the Deadwyler case in connection with the black man who was shot dead by police. The McCone Commission investigation into the Watts riots and their recommendation regarding the community's need for healthcare ultimately led to the construction of the Dr. Martin Luther King, Jr. General Hospital in Watts, California, in 1972 and Martin Luther King, Jr. Multi-Service Ambulatory Care Center in 1972 (which has since been replaced by the Martin Luther King, Jr. Community Hospital, or MLK-LA) in South Central.

From a personal perspective, I viewed these developments as extremely significant in the evolution of a new societal scheme that could revolutionize a dysfunctional healthcare delivery system riddled with racial and ethnic disparities. Inspired by this possibility, I left my position as a member of the faculty of Harvard Medical School and moved from Boston back to Los Angeles to accept an appointment as the assistant medical director at the new hospital, and I was instrumental in its opening in 1972. This gave me an opportunity to observe firsthand the grave health conditions that blacks were struggling against. My close-up view of black health status also allowed me to chronicle the adverse medical conditions affecting blacks, and it gave me the impetus to write the *Textbook of Black-Related Diseases* [15] in 1975. It also inspired me to consider starting a new black healthcare organization focused on cardiovascular disease (CVD), which my research revealed was the number one killer of black Americans rather than homicidal violence or self-inflicted black-on-black crime.

As I moved forward in creating what was to become the ABC, I encountered some resistance to the idea from some of my medical colleagues. Most of this lack of acceptance came primarily from white colleagues who did not seem to have an understanding of the need for such a group; they felt that the wonderful system of cardiovascular care in the United States, the envy of the world, was equally good for whites and blacks. When I pointed out that the Framingham Study [16], a large ongoing clinical investigation of heart disease initiated in 1948 by the National Institutes of Health (NIH), contained no blacks among its 5209 subjects, and that therefore the study findings may not be applicable to blacks, they did not seem to comprehend my conviction that "one size does not fit all" and that approaches to health issues in blacks should be tailored to their characteristics. They gave me the impression that there was no need for me to put any focus on heart disease in blacks. There was also an objection, articulated to me by leaders of the largest of the major heart organizations, that monies collected by them from various sources, including public and private funders, should be utilized almost entirely for basic and clinical research rather than for community benefit (personal communication). This ignorance, lack of recognition, and blindness to the particular needs of blacks was part of my rationale for founding the ABC. It had become obvious to me that cardiovascular care for African Americans was not going to progress unless we established our own organization to define our own priorities and objectives and seized the opportunity to tailor our methods of approaching and eliminating disparities to our particular needs.

This was the rationale for establishing the ABC, which I founded at the annual convention of the American Heart Association (AHA) in Dallas, Texas, in November

1974. It was a purely spontaneous event that was not planned in advance; I organized a dinner meeting involving every black cardiologist I could find in attendance at the AHA convention; 17 physicians sat down with me over dinner to discuss the cardio-vascular crisis confronting African Americans and what we should and could do to deal with it. I suggested the name, Association of Black Cardiologists, which was accepted by consensus by the group, and I was recognized as the Founder and was elected president (Fig. 4.9). The founding members who joined me at that historic meeting were Elijah Saunders, MD; Paul Terry Batiste, MD; Walter M. Booker, Sr., PhD; Daniel D. Savage, MD, PhD; Kermit L. Brown, MD; Charles L. Curry, MD; Major Geer, MD; Richard F. Gillum, MD; L. Julian Haywood, MD; Hannibal E. Howell, MD; Paul M. Jackson, MD; Edith Irby Jones, MD; Alphonzo Jordan, MD; Levi V. Perry, MD; Huerta C. Neals, MD; Boisey O. Barnes, MD; and Felipe Robinson, MD. We decided that our main purpose was to uplift and improve the cardiovascular health of African Americans. And importantly, we wanted to operate in collaboration with other heart organizations rather than in competition with them.

Within a year, the ABC had attracted the attention of the leadership of the AHA, who requested a meeting with me at their headquarters in Dallas, Texas, to explain what we were all about. So I attended that meeting, which consisted of a "who's who" of cardiology in the United States. After reassuring them that our black

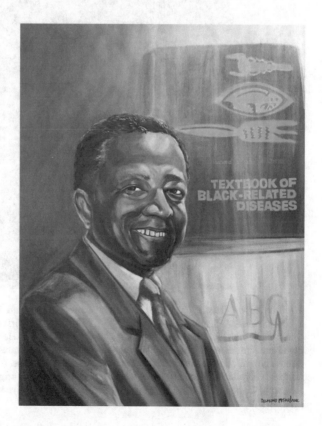

Fig. 4.9 Richard Allen Williams, MD, Founder and the Inaugural President of the Association of Black Cardiologists (ABC) in 1974 and author of the *Textbook of Black-Related Diseases* in 1975, which has been entered into the Smithsonian Institution's National Museum of African American History and Culture. (Portrait by Desmond McFarlane; photograph courtesy of Dr. Williams)

organization was not a militant or "invasive" group (to borrow a term from the cardiology vernacular) set upon destroying the status quo of the AHA or indeed any aspect of cardiology, I appealed to them and spoke truth to power while asking them to help us in our struggle to establish ourselves. This appeal was successful in that they assigned one of their black staffers, Glen Bennett, to be our first Executive Director, with his salary being paid by the AHA. Glen continued in that role for 10 years and worked constantly by my side as we developed our fledgling group.

Over the next few years, we were able to recruit almost every black cardiologist whom we could identify into our ranks, including the few who were enrolled in fellowship training programs, as well as the two most senior African Americans in the field, John Thomas, MD, Chief of Cardiology at Meharry Medical College, and John Beauregard Johnson, MD, Chief of Cardiology at Howard University College of Medicine (Fig. 4.10). During the conventions of the major heart organizations,

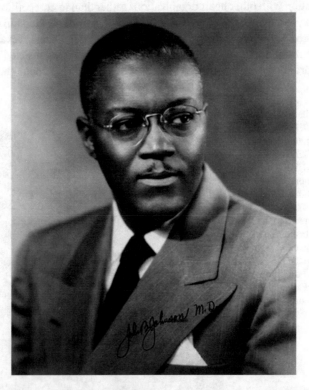

Fig. 4.10 John Beauregard Johnson, MD (1908–1972) (Howard University, Washington DC, 1955; Scurlock, Addison, Photographer. 1883–1964), one of the first black cardiologists, who was Chief of Cardiology at Howard University College of Medicine. He was the first to identify high blood pressure as a serious medical problem for blacks. Unfortunately, he was a victim of the disease himself, and he died suddenly from a cerebral hemorrhage. (Courtesy National Library of Medicine Digital Collection. NLM Unique ID: 101419604; original in Moorland-Spingarn Research Center, Howard University Archives, Howard University, Washington DC, with permission)

we established well-respected scientific sessions that attracted black as well as white cardiologists, and we even served as a role model for the development of cardiovascular-based organizations of other ethnic groups such as the American Association of Cardiologists of Indian Origin (AACIO). Importantly, we were able to influence NIH to initiate an investigation of heart disease in African Americans, which is the ongoing Jackson Heart Study [17] headed for years by the brilliant Herman Taylor, MD. Called the "black Framingham Study" by some, the Jackson Heart Study has gone a long way in correcting many of the misconceptions and providing new insights about cardiovascular disease in blacks. Gary Gibbons, MD, the current director of the National Heart, Lung, and Blood Institute of the NIH and an outstanding researcher in his own right, is collaborating with the ABC and carrying on the new thrust of promoting cardiovascular disease prevention and wellness programs among blacks and other vulnerable subpopulations in the United States.

One of the ABC's main impacts was to stimulate and inspire black medical students to pursue careers in cardiology, where there has always been a dire need for more physicians of color. This was not an easy task, because there was an impression among black students that trying to find cardiology programs that would accept blacks was likely to result in frustration. In fact, the ABC conducted a survey of all cardiology training programs in the country and found that most had never had a black trainee, while a few had several black fellows. We decided that this information should be published in our ABC newsletter, along with what we called the "Hall of Shame" to indicate those programs that did not have blacks. We even singled out the worst offenders, and our Chief Executive Officer at the time, B. Waine Kong, met with them and confronted them. This aggressive effort had excellent results. An example was The Ohio State University, which had never trained a black cardiologist; coincident with our meeting with them, the cardiology chief, Dr. Bill Abraham, decided to make diversity a focus. He hired ABC member Dr. Quinn Capers, IV, and along with other leaders at the institution, they led a vigorous recruitment effort that resulted in their going from "worst to first." They are now one of the most diverse cardiology training programs and cardiology faculties in the nation. Figure 4.11 shows Dr. Quinn Capers, IV, who heads the Interventional Cardiology Fellowship Training Program for The Ohio State University Wexner Medical Center, with cardiology faculty and trainees at Ohio State.

The ABC also created ethnocentric programs involving medical education and clinical research, led by Jay Brown, MD, Michelle Albert, MD, and Eldrin Lewis, MD; heart disease in African American women, an initiative put forward by a rising group of black female cardiologists, including Elizabeth Ofili, MD, and Rosalyn Sterling-Scott, MD; epidemiology, led by Richard Gillum, MD; lipids, led by Karol Watson, MD; nutrition, an initiative led by Shiriki Kumanyika, PhD, and Tazewell Banks, MD, with particular emphasis on the dangers of the soul food diet; special considerations for the pharmacological treatment of blacks, i.e., the use of beta-blockers and ACE inhibitors, which may have different effects on blacks compared to whites due to genetic polymorphisms [18], as well as special aspects of drug research, led by Walter Booker, PhD; hypertension in blacks, led by Elijah Saunders, MD, Keith Ferdinand, MD, and Boisey Barnes, MD; coronary heart disease in blacks, led by Alphonso Jordan, MD, Charles Curry, MD,

Fig. 4.11 Quinn Capers IV, MD, Professor of Medicine, Division of Cardiovascular Medicine, indoor version: (*4th from the right*); with his team of black cardiologists and cardiology fellows at The Ohio State University College of Medicine, Columbus, Ohio, May 2018. (Photograph courtesy of Dr. Capers)

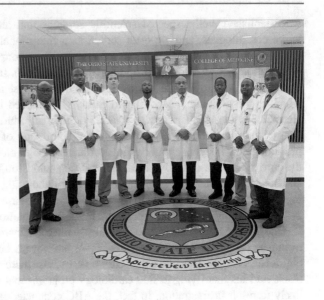

and Julian Haywood, MD; the use of hydralazine and isosorbide dinitrate (BiDil) in blacks with heart failure, led by Ann Taylor, MD [18]; lack of inclusion of blacks in clinical trials, led by Dan Savage, MD; cardiac imaging, led by Kim A. Williams, MD, and Ola Akimboboye, MD; lack of access for blacks to expensive medications and cardiovascular devices such as defibrillators and procedures such as transcatheter aortic valve replacement (TAVR), led by Aaron Horne, MD; electrophysiology, led by Augustus Grant, MD, Roosevelt Gilliam, MD, and John Fontaine, MD; and heart failure, led by Clyde Yancy, MD. All of these programs have been admirably administered by ABC CEO Cassandra McCullough. It also helped to facilitate important cardiovascular research projects, such as the African American Heart Failure Trial (A-HeFT) [19]. This investigation, discussed more fully in Chap. 1, was a significant departure from the conventional thinking that treatment of illnesses such as heart failure should be the same in all people as members of the same species. Some authorities considered that it was tantamount to medical heresy to propose that the response to a drug might be different in different races and even to suggest that there may be differential responses to treatment by race was to intimate a type of reverse racial bias. This was the basis of the controversy that erupted when the A-HeFT Study, conceived by Dr. Jay Cohn, a white cardiologist, and led by principal investigator, Dr. Ann Taylor, a black cardiologist, was conducted in collaboration with the ABC. The basic premise was that a fixed combination of vasodilators, hydralazine, and isosorbide dinitrate would be significantly more effective than an ACE inhibitor in decreasing mortality and morbidity in African American patients suffering from severe heart failure than in a comparative cohort of black patients not receiving this regimen. The hypothesis was proven when the study showed a 43% decrease in mortality in the group receiving the fixed-dose combination, which went on to be marketed as BiDil, a drug designed specifically for the black population of patients with heart failure [20]. There were some detractors who felt that this represented "reverse discrimination" in medicine because the drug did not benefit everyone equally, which has made it appear that blacks were being shown a perverse favoritism because the drug helped them and not whites. I regard this as a spurious, unscientific, anti-intellectual argument that flies in the face of the facts that emerged from an excellent randomized clinical trial.

Conclusion

In this chapter, two examples have been provided of black medical organizations that have advanced the concept that deliberate efforts are necessary to achieve progress in eliminating healthcare disparities; improving medical educational opportunities; increasing cultural competence; and enhancing diversity, inclusion, and equity for African Americans. The most successful efforts have been made at the organizational rather than at the individual or institutional level. These black organizations have served as beacons leading the way for predominately white groups to become more open to the participation and involvement of African Americans in their societies and in organized medicine in general. In this fashion, everyone benefits from collaboration evolving from the social context and translated into clinical gains. The hope is that this precedent continues and increases over time.

References

1. History Matters. The U.S. Survey Course on the Web. Booker T. Washington delivers the 1895 Atlanta compromise speech. American Social History Project/Center for Media and Learning (Graduate Center, CUNY) and the Roy Rosenzweig Center for History and New Media (George Mason University). http://historymatters.gmu.edu/d/39/. Accessed 30 Sep 2019.
2. Penn IG, Bowen JWE. The united Negro: his problems and his progress, containing the addresses and proceedings the Negro young people's Christian and education congress held August 6–11, 1902. Atlanta: De Luther Publishing Co; 1902.
3. The doctor's reading matter. J Natl Med Assoc. 1911;3(1):59–61.
4. Cobb WM. Dr. Daniel Hale Williams 1858–1931. J Natl Med Assoc. 1953;45(5):379–85.
5. Morrison SM, Fee E. The Journal of the National Medical Association: a voice for civil rights and social justice. Am J Public Health. 2010;100(Suppl 1):S70–1.
6. O'Toole P. Theodore Roosevelt cared deeply about the sick. Who knew? The New York Times. Opinion. 6 Jan 2019. https://www.nytimes.com/2019/01/06/opinion/theodore-roosevelt-health-care-progressive.html. Accessed 17 Oct 2019.
7. Morris K. The Founding of the National Medical Association. Yale Medicine Thesis Digital Library. 360; 2007. https://elischolar.library.yale.edu/ymtdl/360.
8. Cobb WM. The first Negro medical society: a history of the Medico-chirurgical Society of the District of Columbia, 1884–1939. Washington, DC: Associated Publishers; 1939. p. 11.
9. Lynk MV. Sixty years of medicine; or, the life and times of Dr. Miles V. Lynk, an autobiography. Memphis: Twentieth Century Press; 1951. p. 1.
10. Byrd WM, Clayton LA. An American health dilemma. (Vol. 1) A medical history of African Americans and the problem of race. Beginnings to 1900. New York: Routledge; 2000. p. 399.
11. Williams RA, editor. Healthcare disparities at the crossroads with healthcare reform. New York: Springer and Business Media; 2011.
12. CNN Politics. Election Center 2008. Transcript: 'This is your victory,' says Obama. http://edition.cnn.com/2008/POLITICS/11/04/obama.transcript/. Accessed 30 Sep 2019.
13. George A. The 1968 Kerner Commission got it right, but nobody listened. Smithsonian. 1 Mar 2018. https://www.smithsonianmag.com/smithsonian-institution/1968-kerner-commission-got-it-right-nobody-listened-180968318/. Accessed 17 Oct 2019.

14. Pyncheon T. A journey into the mind of Watts. The New York Times. Books. 12 June 1966. https://archive.nytimes.com/www.nytimes.com/books/97/05/18/reviews/pynchon-watts.html. Accessed 17 Oct 2019.
15. Williams RA, editor. Textbook of black-related diseases. New York: McGraw-Hill; 1975.
16. Kannel WB. Bishop Lecture. Contribution of the Framingham Study to preventive cardiology. J Am Coll Cardiol. 1990;15(1):206–11.
17. Taylor HA Jr. The Jackson Heart Study: an overview. Ethn Dis. 2005;15(4 Suppl 6):S6-1-3.
18. Burroughs VJ, Maxey RW, Levy RA. Racial and ethnic differences in response to medicines: towards individualized pharmaceutical treatment. J Natl Med Assoc. 2002;94(10 Suppl):1–26.
19. Taylor AL, Ziesche S, Yancy C, Carson P, D'Agostino R Jr, Ferdinand K, et al. African-American Heart Failure Trial Investigators. Combination of isosorbide dinitrate and hydralazine in blacks with heart failure. N Engl J Med. 2004;351(20):2049–57.
20. Arbor Pharmaceuticals (Atlanta GA). Highlights of prescribing information BiDil ©2019. https://www.bidil.com/pdf/bidil-pi.pdf. Accessed 17 Oct 2019.

Healthcare Reform Law (Obamacare): Update on "The Good, the Bad, and the Ugly" and the Persistence of Polarization on Repeal and Replace

5

Introduction

In my 2011 book, *Healthcare Disparities at the Crossroads with Healthcare Reform*, I detailed the Patient Protection and Affordable Care Act, or the ACA, also often referred to as Obamacare, and spoke of it as having good, bad, and frankly ugly characteristics, so regarded according to one's political orientation [1]. Under the "good" aspect, Obamacare might be considered as a blessing that uplifts the health and welfare of mankind and accomplishes the "Triple Aim" of healthcare reform: (a) provision of greater access to healthcare for the American people; (b) lowering the costs of medical treatment; and (c) increasing the quality of healthcare delivery. Under the "bad" rubric, it may be thought of as a well-intended piece of legislation that is incomplete in that it does not provide universal coverage of the American population. Under the "ugly" title, it might be seen by its Republican detractors as a downright danger to the public in not providing the promised high standard of healthcare and in being too expensive. In this chapter, we will examine the progress made in reforming healthcare delivery in the United States, and we will briefly consider the pros and cons of Obamacare and the attempts that are being made to repeal, replace, augment, change, and improve it.

The Backdrop for Current Healthcare Reform Efforts

This chapter is being written during a turbulent, uncertain time in the history of health reform and indeed in politics in general in the United States. The backdrop is the situation created by the Presidential election on November 8, 2016, in which Republican Donald Trump won the contest over Democrat Hillary Clinton. Mr. Trump vowed to repeal the ACA or Obamacare promulgated by President Barack Obama on his first day in office, which was January 21, 2017. Despite the fact that he was warned that there is no replacement that had been approved and that such an act would jeopardize the health and lives of almost 30 million people who would be

© Springer Nature Switzerland AG 2020
R. A. Williams, *Blacks in Medicine*, https://doi.org/10.1007/978-3-030-41960-8_5

deprived of health insurance coverage, he was determined to persist. In fact, even if there was a replacement plan, there would be no money to pay for it, because the cost to the economy of repealing the ACA would be about $350 billion dollars over the next 10 years, based on Congressional Budget Office (CBO) data.

The accomplishments of the ACA over the almost 10 years since its passage and being signed into law on March 23, 2010 are numerous and have been presented in great detail in an article by none other than President Obama, the first sitting president to write a scholarly paper for a peer-reviewed medical journal [2]. There was a documented increased access to care, with the uninsured rate declining by a huge 43 percent, from 16.0 in 2010 to 9.1 in 2017. The first graph in the Obama article (not shown here; gain open access to full article via https://jamanetwork.com/journals/jama/fullarticle/2533698) provides a stark comparison of the uninsured rates over time from prior to the creation of Medicare and Medicaid through 2015 and indicates the dramatic impact that the ACA had after its coverage provisions took effect. Accordingly, 20 million people who were previously uninsured received health insurance coverage by 2017, and that improvement has been maintained. Medicare spending has been reduced, and Medicare is projected to spend 20% or $160 billion less in 2019 alone, as projected by the non-partisan CBO. In the arena of quality of care improvements, the Agency for Healthcare Research and Quality (AHRQ) estimates that the decline in conditions acquired in hospitals has saved 84,000 lives over a 4-year period. Thus, it appears that material gains have accrued from the ACA in all components of the Triple Aim of healthcare reform.

Beyond the fiscal impact that repeal would have, we must contend with the potential human tragedy associated with "de-insuring" 20–30 million citizens whose medical security depends on Obamacare. Specifically, repeal would increase the uninsured in our population by 23 million. When one considers the gains that were made in insurance coverage through application of Obamacare and expanded Medicaid, which is operative in 36 states and the District of Columbia, via which three million blacks and four million Hispanics achieved coverage, repeal is certain to cause a "whiplash" effect if this healthcare security system is withdrawn. The uninsured rates that plunged 11.8% for blacks and 11.3% for Hispanics compared to a 7.3% drop for white non-Hispanics since the inception of Obamacare in 2010 (2016 report from the Office of the Assistant Secretary for Planning and Evaluation, Department of Health and Human Services) are expected to go back to the levels that existed previously. Thus, blacks and other minorities who benefited from a reduction of healthcare disparities as a direct result of the ACA now stand to suffer disproportionately from its withdrawal. Although the ACA has its imperfections and problems, these are far less negatively impactful from a health standpoint than what will occur if the ACA is removed. If that occurs, it is possible to foresee dire consequences, especially for blacks and other racial and ethnic minorities.

It has been a decade since the ACA was signed into law, and since the very beginning of the Trump administration, political and legal challenges have been levied against it. Although most of these challenges have been turned back, there has recently been a very significant action by a federal appellate court that threatens the ACA's survival more than any previous action. On December 14, 2018, Judge Reed

O'Connor, a US District Court judge, ruled that the ACA was unconstitutional. This ruling was based on the case of *Texas v. Azar*, which was brought by the Republican attorneys general of 20 states who contended that since the ACA's individual mandate, which penalized individuals who did not purchase health insurance, had been eliminated in 2017 and therefore was no longer constitutional, the entire law was not viable and was itself unconstitutional. In agreeing with the Republican plaintiffs, Judge O'Connor subsequently struck down all provisions that were previously made under the ACA, including insurance regulations, subsidies, expansion of Medicaid, reforms of Medicare, and other measures. In response, 21 Democratic attorneys general representing 21 states have appealed Judge O'Connor's ruling to the US Court of Appeals for the Fifth Circuit. The Trump administration's response to this appeal was to have the Justice Department, on March 25, 2019, request the invalidation of the entire ACA and to affirm Judge O'Connor's ruling.

Thus, at this time, the ACA sits in limbo awaiting an appeals court decision [3]. In a very real sense, the medical fate of millions of citizens rests in the hands of judges and politicians rather than physicians. Although there have been speculations by legal scholars [4] that the Fifth Circuit will overturn Judge O'Connor's decision and that in any case, if the issue goes to the Supreme Court, he will not prevail, there is still concern. And President Trump's plans to pass yet another Republican alternative to the ACA is being given no chance by political pundits who think that the mid-term Congressional elections of 2018, which swept several Republican ACA opponents out of office and replaced them with Democrats, creating a Democrat-controlled House of Delegates, have made it impossible for repeal to occur.

However, that does not necessarily provide solace for those who are in favor of retaining the ACA, because many Democrat lawmakers now see some glaring weaknesses in the law and are advocating that a new structure, called Medicare for All, should replace it.

The Most Recent Thinking on Healthcare Reform

Among Democrats, there are two schools of thought about what shape healthcare reform should take. The more conservative view is that the ACA should be maintained in its basic form but that its inadequacies should be fixed. In other words, repair it, don't replace it. The rationale of this group is that replacement would mean losing certain popular features such as the pre-existing conditions provision, which mandates that insurers must cover patients for conditions that pre-date their subscription to health insurance. This group is also encouraged by the fact that Medicaid expansion is gaining acceptance among more states such as Louisiana, which now has a Democrat as Governor, bringing the current number up to 36 states and the District of Columbia. This group is also hopeful that a bipartisan compromise can be worked out to revise Obamacare in a manner that will be acceptable to both sides. The liberal view encompasses those who feel that bipartisan collaboration is unlikely in the current highly polarized Congressional atmosphere [5] and that, in any event, the ACA will never provide truly universal care.

Several Democrats are of the opinion that the nation would be better off adopting a single-payer plan called Medicare for All, which would be much more inclusive of the American public. Figure 5.1 is a comparison between the Single-Payer Bill H.R. 676, the Affordable Care Act, and the American Health Care Act (the ill-fated Republican "repeal and replace" plan) according to the Physicians for a National Health Program.

Medicare for All may be further defined as a system in which a single public or quasi-public agency organizes healthcare financing, but the delivery of the health-care remains largely in private hands. All US residents would be covered for all medically necessary services, including physician, hospital, preventive, long-term care, mental health, reproductive, dental, vision, prescription drug, and medical supply costs (from Physicians for a National Health Program). Theoretically, this would be a system of universal care for the United States, the only highly developed country in the world without it. Fifty-one other countries have it, from Norway to Kuwait.

There is a great deal of controversy currently about the cost of such a system, which has been estimated to be in the trillions of dollars in the next decade, and about the source of the funding for it. One suggested source of funding is new taxes,

A Comparison: Single-Payer Legislation vs. Affordable Care Act vs. American Health Care Act			
	Single-Payer Bill, H.R. 676	**Affordable Care Act (ACA)**	**American Health Care Act**
Universal Coverage	**Yes.** Everyone is covered automatically at birth.	**No.** About 28 million will still be uninsured in 2022 and tens of millions will remain underinsured, i.e. facing obstacles to access and at risk of financial hardship if they get seriously ill.	**No.** The Congressional Budget Office estimates 14 million (additional) people would lose insurance in the first year alone. By 2026, 24 million would lose coverage, leading to a total of 52 million uninsured in that year.
Full Range of Benefits	**Yes.** Coverage for all medically necessary care, including inpatient and outpatient services, prescription drugs, dental, vision, and long-term care.	**No.** Insurers continue to strip down policies (leaving many services uncovered) and increase patients' premiums, co-payments and deductibles.	**No.** Insurers continue to strip down policies (leaving even more services uncovered in "catastrophic" plans, e.g.) and increase patients' premiums, co-payments and deductibles.
Savings	**Yes.** Redirects $500 billion in administrative waste to care, resulting in first-dollar coverage and no net increase in U.S. health spending.	**No.** Increases health spending by about $1.1 trillion over 10 years. Adds further layers of administrative bloat to our health system through the introduction of state-based exchanges.	**Some,** but mainly for wealthy taxpayers. The CBO says the AHCA would reduce the federal deficit by $150 billion over nine years, largely by eliminating federal payouts to Medicaid and subsidies. Taxes on the wealthy that help fund health services would decrease.
Cost Control & Sustainability	**Yes.** Large-scale cost controls (negotiated fee schedule with physicians, bulk purchasing of drugs, hospital budgeting, capital planning, etc.) ensure that benefits are sustainable over the long term.	**No.** Preserves a fragmented system incapable of controlling costs. Gains in coverage are erased by rising out-of-pocket expenses, bureaucratic waste and profiteering by private insurers and Big Pharma.	**No.** Preserves a fragmented system incapable of controlling costs. Out-of-pocket expenses will continue to rise, as will bureaucratic waste and profiteering by private insurers and Big Pharma.
Choice of Doctor & Hospital	**Yes.** Patients are allowed free choice of their doctor and hospital.	**No.** Insurance companies continue to deny and limit care and to maintain restrictive networks.	**No.** Insurance companies continue to deny and limit care and to maintain restrictive networks.
Progressive Financing	**Yes.** Premiums and out-of-pocket costs are replaced with progressive income and wealth taxes. 95 percent of American households will pay less for care than they do now.	**No.** Continues the unfair financing of health care whereby costs are disproportionately paid by paid by middle- and lower-income Americans and those families facing acute or chronic illness.	**No.** Continues and aggravates, via new, inequitable tax credits, the unfair financing of health care whereby costs are disproportionately paid by middle- and lower-income Americans and families facing acute or chronic illness.

PHYSICIANS FOR A NATIONAL HEALTH PROGRAM   www.pnhp.org | info@pnhp.org

Fig. 5.1 Comparison between Single-Payer Bill H.R. 676, the Affordable Care Act, and the American Health Care Act (the ill-fated Republican "repeal and replace" plan). (Courtesy, Physicians for a National Health Program, with permission)

which would presumably be imposed on the rich. Another area of controversy is whether private insurance coverage would be eliminated or at least diminished. The debate over whether it should be put forth as a replacement for Obamacare promises to continue into the 2020 elections and beyond.

Conclusion

At this point, it is impossible to predict what type of healthcare reform measures will emerge from the intense debate and controversy that are going on. The outcome of court deliberations and Congressional action is critical to the health and welfare of the American people, and particularly to minority group citizens. To a great extent, the people themselves are in a position to help determine the outcome according to the way they vote in the next national election; they already have taken some steps in that direction in the mid-term election of 2018, when the Democrats achieved a majority in the House of Representatives. It is obvious that the most significant healthcare crisis in US history will depend on political decisions. It is also certain that we cannot as a nation continue to "kick the (healthcare reform) can down the road," as was done in the past beginning in 1910 when President Teddy Roosevelt attempted unsuccessfully to pass a viable bill, up to 2010 when President Barack Obama did so successfully. We must now build upon the documented gains that have accrued from Obamacare. The final form that the system takes will ultimately be decided by the American people, probably with input from the US Supreme Court.

References

1. Williams RA, editor. Healthcare disparities at the crossroads with healthcare reform. New York: Springer and Business Media; 2011.
2. Obama B. United States health care reform. Progress to date and next steps. JAMA. 2016;316(5):525–32.
3. Oberlander J. Sitting in limbo—Obamacare under divided government. N Engl J Med. 2019;380(26):2485–7.
4. Jost TS. Court decision to invalidate the Affordable Care Act would affect every American. 17 Dec 2018. New York: The Commonwealth Fund. To the Point. https://www.commonwealth-fund.org/blog/2018/court-decision-invalidate-affordable-care-act-would-affect-every-american. Accessed 30 Sep 2019.
5. Binder SA. Polarized we govern? 27 May 2014. Washington, DC: Brookings Institution. Series: Strengthening American Democracy. https://www.brookings.edu/research/polarized-we-govern/. Accessed 30 Sep 2019.

Outstanding Black Physicians and Other Health Professionals in American History

6

> *Where there is no vision, the people perish.*
>
> —Proverbs 29:18 KJV

It is axiomatic that any attempt to create a list of the best or most important or most accomplished people in any field will be met with questions about why certain individuals were excluded or, indeed, why some were even included. No list of this type will ever satisfy everyone. However, the thought is often raised about who the outstanding physicians are and were, and it certainly is pertinent in a book on blacks in medicine. We sometimes refer to prominent physicians in terms of their demonstrated ability to overcome adversity while accomplishing enormous gains in their careers, against all odds in many cases.

What metrics should we employ to determine who should be on this select list? Often the term "great" is used to describe an individual physician's attributes. However, if greatness can be defined as extraordinary competence sustained over time, many of those who had only a relatively brief opportunity to demonstrate their expertise would not make the list, although their singular accomplishment may have been groundbreaking. So perhaps a broader criterion should be used, one that does not require a long-term application of medical prowess. I would like to suggest what that overarching criterion should be: *it is the unequivocal impact that an individual physician has had in saving and rescuing the lives and health of African American and other minority, vulnerable, needy, and impoverished people, and contributing in a measurable manner to their health and well-being, either by involvement as a medical practitioner, researcher, educator, or academic standout or through leadership and activism as a champion for social justice.* This is a yardstick that is long enough to qualify those who are truly deserving of such recognition but narrow enough to invoke an important amount of exclusivity.

© Springer Nature Switzerland AG 2020
R. A. Williams, *Blacks in Medicine*, https://doi.org/10.1007/978-3-030-41960-8_6

Who should decide and judge who is admitted to this exclusive "Hall of Fame" or pantheon of the best black physicians of all time? Several lists have been offered in the past by a variety of authors; I believe that all have had merit, but all have raised complaints of being too exclusive or unfair. In this instance, I will take the responsibility of putting forth my own list, which is based upon the tenets articulated above. I realize that it may not contain the names of all who should be so honored, but in its defense, let me explain that it is not my intention to be all-inclusive, which is impossible in any event. I simply want to make certain that the majority of those whom I have determined, based on my research, are deserving are represented here, so that the worthy deeds of so many African American physicians and their exploits do not continue to be unrecognized. This is also not a final list by any means; obviously, there can be additions as time goes by, and, judging by the outstanding accomplishments that they have made over the past 400 years in assisting in and protecting the very survival of the black race, their proud tradition will continue into the future. That is the true legacy of blacks in medicine.

Past Presidents of the National Medical Association (NMA)

(Profiles and photographs are based on available information and permissions provided by families and other sources)

1. Robert Fulton Boyd, MD, DDS (1855–1912) (Fig. 6.1) Undergraduate: Fisk University, Nashville, TN. Medical and dental school: Central Tennessee College, Nashville, TN. Physician, dentist, and professor of gynecology and clinical medicine at Meharry Medical College, Nashville, Tennessee. Founder of Mercy Hospital, Nashville, the largest hospital in the South to be owned and managed by African Americans. In his published paper, "What Are the Causes of the Great Mortality Among Negroes in the Cities of the South, and How is That Mortality to be Lessened?" he made some of the earliest and most astute observations regarding the physical condition of Afro-Americans. Along with ten others, he organized a national fraternity of black doctors, the Society of Colored Physicians and Surgeons, of which he was elected president. This group eventually became the National Medical Association [1, 2]. NMA President, 1895–1897.
2. H.T. Noel, MD. NMA President, 1898–1900.
3. O.D. Porter, MD. NMA President, 1901–1902.
4. F.A. Stewart, MD. NMA President, 1903.
5. Charles Victor Roman, MD (1864–1934) (Fig. 6.2). Medical school: Meharry Medical College. Postgraduate: Post-Graduate Medical School and Hospital of Chicago, Chicago, Illinois and the Royal Ophthalmic Hospital and Central London Ear, Nose, and Throat Hospital in London, England. Founder and first head of the Department of Ophthalmology and Otolaryngology at Meharry, serving also as professor of medical history and ethics. First editor of the *Journal of the National Medical Association*. Articulated the theme and

Fig. 6.1 Robert Fulton Boyd, MD, DDS. (From a 1902 book, https://www.worldcat.org/title/twentieth-century-negro-literature-or-a-cyclopedia-of-thought-on-the-vital-topics-relating-to-the-american-negro-by-one-hundred-of-americas-greatest-negroes/oclc/974669349?referer=di&ht=edition, via Project Gutenberg ebook version https://www.gutenberg.org/files/18772/18772-h/18772-h.htm#Page_215, Public Domain, https://commons.wikimedia.org/w/index.php?curid=76659470)

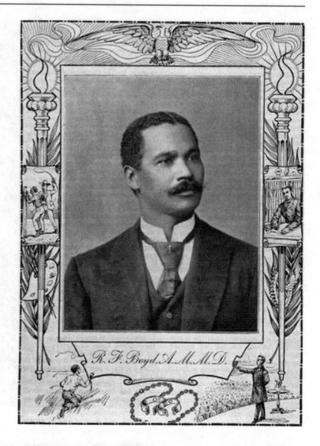

mission of the NMA in 1911, helping to stabilize the fledgling organization [2, 3]. NMA President, 1904.

6. John E. Hunter, MD. NMA President, 1905.
7. R.E. Jones, MD. NMA President, 1906.
8. Nathan Francis Mossell, MD (1856–1946) (Fig. 6.3). Undergraduate: Lincoln University, Philadelphia, PA. Medical school: University of Pennsylvania, Philadelphia. Internship: Guy's, Queen's, and St. Thomas' hospitals, London, UK. Founder, medical director, and chief of staff of the Frederick Douglass Memorial Hospital and Training School for Nurses, Philadelphia, Pennsylvania, served as its medical director for 37 years. Founder of the Philadelphia Branch of the National Association for the Advancement of Colored People (NAACP) and co-founder of the Philadelphia Academy of Medicine and Allied Sciences [4, 5]. NMA President, 1907.
9. W.H. Wright, MD. NMA President, 1908.
10. P.A. Johnson, MD. NMA President, 1909.
11. Marcus F. Wheatland, MD. NMA President, 1910.
12. Austin M. Curtis, MD. NMA President, 1911.
13. H.F. Gamble, MD. NMA President, 1912.

Fig. 6.2 Charles Victor
Roman, MD. (© Special
Collections and Archives,
Tennessee State University,
with permission)

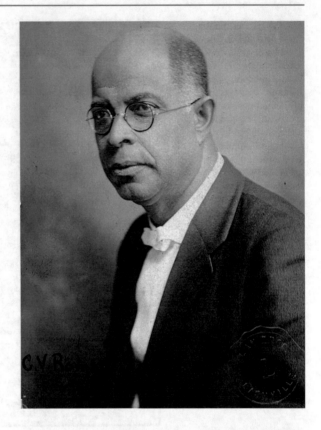

Fig. 6.3 Nathan Francis
Mossell, MD (Unknown -
The Crisis (Jan 1912),
p. 120, Public Domain,
https://commons.
wikimedia.org/w/index.
php?curid=69394930)

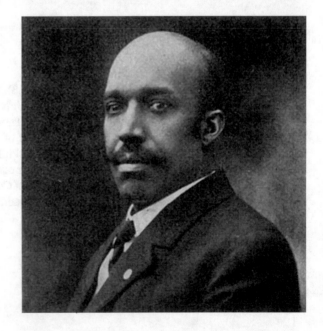

14. John A. Kenny, Sr., MD. NMA President, 1913.
15. A.M. Brown, MD. NMA President, 1914.
16. F.S. Hargraves, MD. NMA President, 1915.
17. Ulysses Grant Dailey, MD. NMA President, 1916.
18. D.W. Byrd, MD. NMA President, 1917.
19. George W. Cabaniss, MD. NMA President, 1918.
20. D.A. Ferguson, DDS. NMA President, 1919.
21. J.W. Jones, MD, NMA President, 1920.
22. John P. Turner, MD. NMA President, 1921.
23. H.M. Green, MD. NMA President, 1922.
24. J. Edward Perry, MD. NMA President, 1923.
25. John O. Plummer, MD. NMA President, 1924.
26. Michael Q. Dumas, MD. NMA President, 1925.
27. Walter G. Alexander, MD. NMA President, 1926.
28. Carl G. Roberts, MD. NMA President, 1927.
29. C.V. Freeman, DDS. NMA President, 1928.
30. T. Spotuas Burwell, MD. NMA President, 1929.
31. L.A. West, MD, NMA President, 1930.
32. W.H. Higgins, MD. NMA President, 1931.
33. Peter M. Murray, MD. NMA President, 1932.
34. C. Hamilton Francis, MD. NMA President, 1933.
35. Midian O. Bousfield, MD. NMA President, 1934.
36. John H. Hale, MD. NMA President, 1935.
37. W. Harry Barnes, MD. NMA President, 1936.
38. Roscoe C. Giles, MD. NMA President, 1937.
39. Lyndon M. Hill, MD. NMA President, 1938.
40. George W. Bowles, MD. NMA President, 1939.
41. Albert W. Dumas, Sr., MD. NMA President, 1940.
42. Kenneth W. Clement, MD. NMA President, 1941.
43. Arthur M. Vaughn, MD. NMA President, 1942.
44. Henry Eugene Lee, MD. NMA President, 1943.
45. T. Manuel Smith, MD. NMA President, 1944–1945.
46. Emory I. Robinson, MD. NMA President, 1946.
47. Walter M. Young, MD. NMA President, 1947.
48. J.A.C. Lattimore, MD. NMA President, 1948.
49. C. Austin Whittier, MD. NMA President, 1949.
50. C. Herbert Marshall, MD. NMA President, 1950.
51. Henry H. Walker, MD. NMA President, 1951.
52. Joseph G. Gathings, MD. NMA President, 1952.
53. Witter C. Atkinson, MD. NMA President, 1953.
54. Porter Davis, MD. NMA President, 1954.
55. Matthew Walker, MD. NMA President, 1955.
56. A.C. Terrence, MD. NMA President, 1956.
57. T.R.M. Howard, MD. NMA President, 1957.
58. Arthur M. Townsend, Jr., MD. NMA President, 1958.

59. R. Stillman Smith, MD. NMA President, 1959.
60. Edward C. Mazique, MD (1911–1987). Undergraduate: Morehouse College, Atlanta, GA. Medical school: Howard University College of Medicine, Washington, DC. Postgraduate: Internship and residency, Freedmen's Hospital, Internal Medicine. Master of Education (MEd), Atlanta University. Past President, Medico-Chirurgical Society of the District of Columbia. Former member and medical staff, Georgetown University Hospital and Providence Hospital. Chaired the Health Services Coordination Committee for the Poor People's Campaign March on Washington in 1968. NMA President, 1960.
61. James T. Aldrich, MD. NMA President, 1961.
62. Vaughn C. Mason, MD. NMA President, 1962.
63. John A. Kenney, Jr., MD. NMA President, 1963.
64. W. Montague Cobb, MD, PhD (1904–1990) (Fig. 6.4). Undergraduate: Amherst College, Amherst, MA. Medical school: Howard University College of Medicine. Postgraduate: PhD in Anatomy and Anthropology, Western Reserve University, Cleveland, OH. Chair, Department of Anatomy (1947–1969), and the first to be named a distinguished professor at Howard University. Principal historian of the African American in medicine and editor of the *Journal of the National Medical Association* (1950–1977). Engaged in the struggle for civil rights and for improved medical care for African Americans, as well as racial integration of hospitals. Lobbied for the passage of Medicare-Medicaid legislation. President, NAACP 1976–1982 [6]. NMA President, 1964.

Fig. 6.4 W. Montague Cobb, MD, PhD. (Courtesy National Library of Medicine Digital Collection. NLM Unique ID: 101412157; with kind permission from the Cobb family)

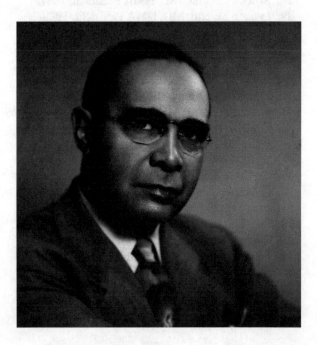

65. Leonidas H. Berry, MD. NMA President, 1965.
66. John L.S. Holloman, Jr., MD. NMA President, 1966.
67. Lionel F. Swann, MD. NMA President, 1967.
68. James M. Whittico, Jr., MD. NMA President, 1968.
69. Julius W. Hill, MD. NMA President, 1969.
70. W.T. Armstrong, MD. NMA President, 1970.
71. Emerson C. Walden, Sr., MD. NMA President, 1971.
72. Edmund C. Casey, MD. NMA President, 1972.
73. Emery L. Rann, MD. NMA President, 1973.
74. Vernal G. Cave, MD. NMA President, 1974.
75. Jasper F. Williams, MD. NMA President, 1975.
76. Arthur H. Coleman, MD. NMA President, 1976.
77. Charles C. Bookert, MD. NMA President, 1977.
78. Jesse B. Barber, Jr., MD. NMA President, 1978.
79. Robert E. Dawson, MD. NMA President, 1979.
80. Vertis R. Thompson, MD. NMA President, 1980.
81. Frank S. Royal, Sr., MD (Fig. 6.5). Undergraduate: Virginia Union University, Richmond, VA. Medical school: Meharry Medical College. Specialty: Family

Fig. 6.5 Frank S. Royal, Sr., MD. (Photograph courtesy of Dr. Royal)

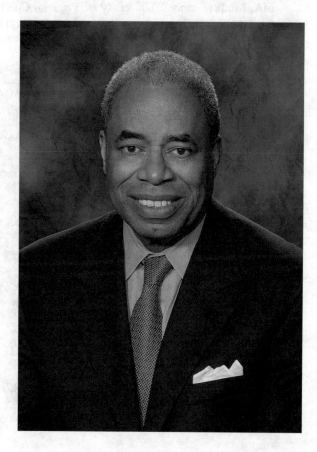

medicine. Assistant Clinical Professor of Family Medicine, Medical College of Virginia, Richmond, VA. Private practice, Bon Secours Health System. NMA President, 1981.

82. Robert L. M. Hilliard, MD. NMA President, 1982.
83. Lucius C. Earles, III, MD. NMA President, 1983.
84. Phillip M. Smith, MD. NMA President, 1984.
85. Edith Irby Jones, MD (1927–2019) (Fig. 6.6). Undergraduate: Knoxville College, Knoxville, TN. Medical school: University of Arkansas School of Medicine, Little Rock (first black student). Specialty: Internal medicine/cardiology. Only female founding member, Association of Black Cardiologists (ABC). Two international healthcare centers bear her name: Dr. Edith Irby Jones Clinic in Vaudreuil, Haiti, which she helped found in 1991, and the Dr. Edith Irby Jones Emergency Clinic in Veracruz, Mexico. NMA President, 1985 (first female President).
86. John O. Brown, MD. NMA President, 1986.
87. John M. Joyner, MD. NMA President, 1987.
88. Frank E. Staggers, Sr., MD. NMA President, 1988.
89. Vivian W. Pinn, MD (Fig. 6.7). Undergraduate: Wellesley College, Wellesley, MA. Medical school: University of Virginia, Charlottesville, VA (the only woman/minority in her class). Postgraduate training: Harvard Medical School,

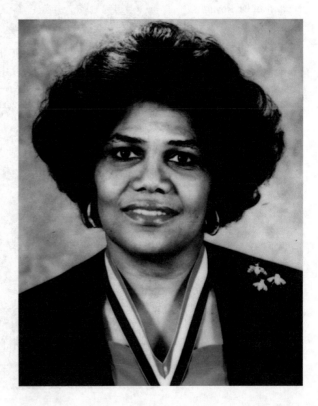

Fig. 6.6 Edith Irby Jones, MD. (Photograph courtesy of the National Medical Association)

Fig. 6.7 Vivian W. Pinn, MD. (Photograph courtesy of Dr. Pinn)

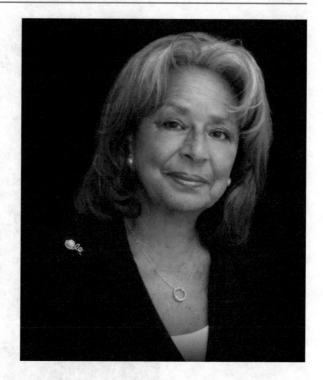

Boston, MA. Specialty: Pathology. Associate Professor of Pathology and Assistant Dean of Student Affairs at Tufts; Professor and Chair Department of Pathology, Howard University College of Medicine. Founding Director, Office of Research on Women's Health, National Institutes of Health (NIH); Senior Scientist Emerita, Fogarty International Center, NIH. Fellow of the American Academy of Arts and Sciences and the National Academy of Medicine. Chair of the NMA Past Presidents' Council (PPC). NMA President, 1989.

90. Charles Johnson, MD (Fig. 6.8). Undergraduate: Howard University. Medical school: Howard University College of Medicine. Specialty: Endocrinology. Professor of Medicine Emeritus, Duke University. Served in the US Air Force as a fighter pilot. NMA President, 1990.

91. Alma Rose George, MD. NMA President, 1991.

92. Richard O. Butcher, MD. NMA President, 1992.

93. Leonard E. Lawrence, MD (Fig. 6.9). Undergraduate: Indiana University. Medical school: Indiana University School of Medicine, Indianapolis. Specialty: Psychiatry/child psychiatry. Emeritus Professor, University of Texas—UT Health San Antonio. NMA President, 1993.

94. Tracy Matthew Walton, Jr., MD (1931–2018) (Fig. 6.10). Undergraduate: Morgan State College, Baltimore, MD. Medical school: Howard University College of Medicine. Specialty: Radiology. Served in over 25 academic and professional capacities and community programs. Held every office in the NMA. NMA President, 1994.

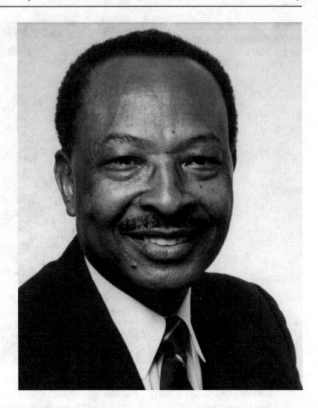

Fig. 6.8 Charles Johnson, MD. (Photograph courtesy of the National Medical Association)

95. Yvonnecris Smith Veal, MD (Fig. 6.11). Undergraduate: Hampton Institute, Hampton, VA. Medical school: Medical College of Virginia. Specialties: Occupational medicine and pediatrics. Former Senior Medical Director, Eastern Region, US Postal Service; former Attending Physician, Pediatrics and Cardiology, Downstate Medical Center. NMA President, 1995.

96. Randall C. Morgan, MD, MBA (Fig. 6.12). Undergraduate: Grinnell College, Grinnell, IA. Medical school: Howard University College of Medicine. Postgraduate: Master of Business Administration (MBA), University of South Florida, Tampa. Specialty: Orthopedic surgery. Executive Director, W. Montague Cobb/NMA Health Institute. Clinical Assistant Professor of Orthopedic Surgery, Florida State University, Tallahassee. Clinical Associate Professor of Orthopedic Surgery, Emeritus, Indiana University School of Medicine. NMA President, 1996.

97. Nathaniel H. Murdock, MD. NMA President, 1997.

98. Gary C. Dennis, MD (Fig. 6.13). Undergraduate: Boston University, Boston, MA. Medical school: Howard University College of Medicine. Postgraduate: Training in Neurosurgery, Baylor College of Medicine, Houston, TX. Past Associate Professor and Former Chief, Division of Neurosurgery, Howard University. Past President, Medical Society of the District of Columbia. NMA President, 1998.

Fig. 6.9 Leonard
E. Lawrence,
MD. (Photograph courtesy
of Dr. Lawrence)

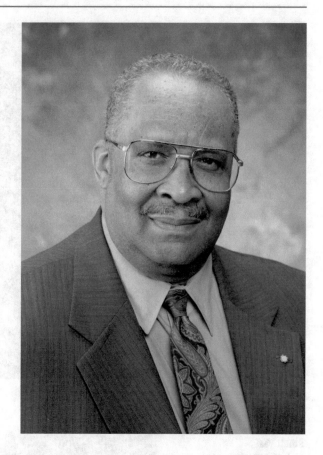

99. Walter W. Shervington, MD. NMA President, 1999. Died in 2000 while serving his term.
100. Javette C. Orgain, MD, MPH (Fig. 6.14). Undergraduate: University of Illinois Chicago. Medical school: University of Illinois at Chicago. Postgraduate: Master of Public Health (MPH), University of Illinois School of Public Health. Specialty: Family medicine. Associate Professor, Department of Family Medicine, University of Illinois at Chicago. Former Assistant Dean of the Urban Health Program, University of Illinois at Chicago College of Medicine. NMA President, 1999 (completed Dr. Shervington's term).
101. Rodney G. Hood, MD, (Fig. 6.15) Undergraduate: Northeastern University School of Pharmacy, Boston, MA. Medical school: University of California (UC) San Diego School of Medicine. Specialty: Internal medicine. Founder and President, Multicultural Healthcare Foundation. CEO, Careview Medical Group. Assistant Clinical Professor of Medicine, UCSD. Editorial Board, *Journal of Racial and Ethnic Health Disparities*. Commissioner and Chair, San Diego Gang Commission for Prevention and Intervention. NMA President, 2000.

Fig. 6.10 Tracy Matthew
Walton, Jr.,
MD. (Photograph courtesy
of the National Medical
Association)

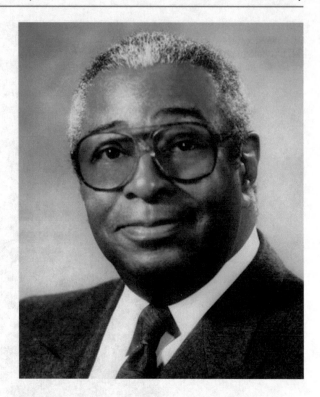

Fig. 6.11 Yvonnecris
Smith Veal
MD. (Photograph courtesy
of the National Medical
Association)

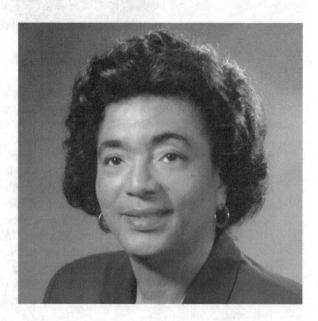

Fig. 6.12 Randall
C. Morgan, Jr., MD,
MBA. (Photograph
courtesy of Dr. Morgan)

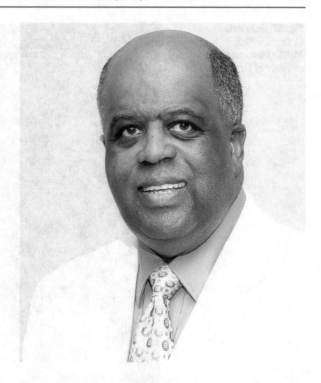

Fig. 6.13 Gary C. Dennis,
MD. (Photograph courtesy
of Dr. Dennis)

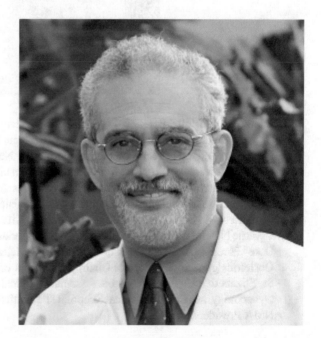

Fig. 6.14 Javette
C. Orgain, MD,
MPH. (Photograph
courtesy of Dr. Orgain)

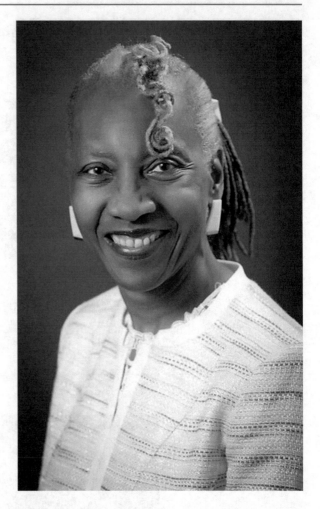

102. Lucille C. Norville Perez, MD (Fig. 6.16). Undergraduate: Manhattanville
     College. Medical school: New York Medical College, Purchase, NY. Specialty:
     Pediatrics and adolescent medicine. Formerly, National Health Director,
     NAACP; Associate Director of the Center for Substance Abuse Prevention at
     the Substance Abuse and Mental Health Services Administration at the US
     Department of Health and Human Services; Assistant Professor of Clinical
     Pediatrics, Mt. Sinai Medical Center, New York City. NMA President, 2001.
103. Laverne Natalie Carroll, MD (Fig. 6.17). Undergraduate: Lake Forest College,
     Lake Forest, IL. Medical school: Meharry Medical College. Specialty:
     Obstetrics/gynecology. Former Chair, Department of Obstetrics/Gynecology,
     St. Elizabeth's Hospital, Houston. Associate Clinical Professor of Obstetrics/
     Gynecology, McGovern Medical School, UT Health Science Center, Houston.
     NMA President, 2002.

Fig. 6.15 Rodney
G. Hood, MD. (Photograph
courtesy of the National
Medical Association)

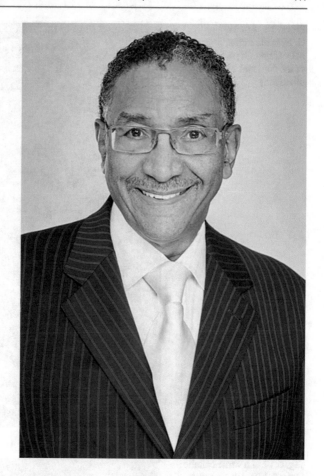

104. Randall W. Maxey, MD, PhD (Fig. 6.18) Undergraduate: University of
     Cincinnati, Ohio. Medical school: Howard University College of Medicine.
     Postgraduate: Residency, Harlem Hospital, Internal Medicine; Fellowship,
     State University of NY (SUNY) Downstate Medical Center, Nephrology;
     PhD, Cardiovascular Pharmacology, Howard University College of Medicine.
     Specialty: Internal medicine/nephrology. Formerly, Assistant Professor of
     Medicine, SUNY Downstate. Alumnus of the Year, Howard University
     College of Medicine, 2002. CEO, Biometrics Management Services. Founder,
     Chairman, and CEO, American Dialysis Holdings. NMA President, 2003.
105. Winston Price, MD (Fig. 6.19). Undergraduate: Brooklyn College of
     CUNY. Medical school: Cornell University Medical College (Weill Cornell
     Medicine, New York). Specialty: Pediatrics. Chief of Staff, Memorial Hospital
     and Manor, Bainbridge, GA. President and Chair, National African American
     Drug Policy Coalition. Clinical Dean, American University of Antigua. NMA
     President, 2004.

Fig. 6.16 Lucille
C. Norville Perez,
MD. (Photograph courtesy
of the National Institutes
of Health)

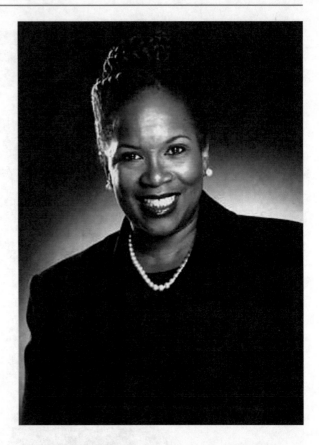

Fig. 6.17 LaVerne Natalie
Carroll, MD. (Photograph
courtesy of the National
Medical Association)

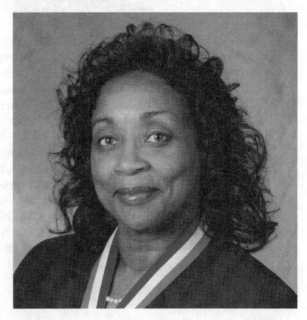

Fig. 6.18 Randall
W. Maxey, MD,
PhD. (Photograph courtesy
of the National Medical
Association)

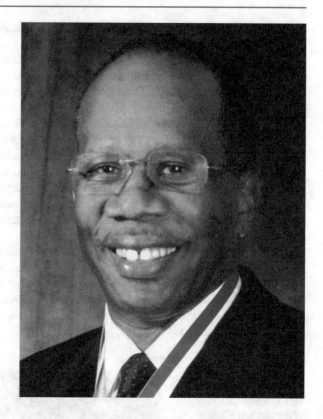

Fig. 6.19 Winston Price,
MD. (Photograph courtesy
of Dr. Price)

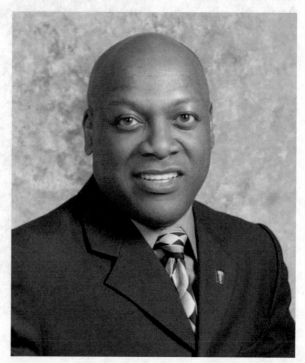

106. Sandra L. Gadson, MD (Fig. 6.20). Undergraduate: Hampton University, Hampton, VA. Medical school: Meharry Medical College. Specialty: Internal medicine/nephrology. Assistant Professor, Internal Medicine, Indiana University. Nephrology Associates of Northern Indiana. NMA President, 2005.
107. Albert W. Morris Jr., MD (Fig. 6.21). Undergraduate: Howard University. Medical school: Howard University College of Medicine. Specialty: Radiology. Diagnostic radiologist (retired), US Department of Veterans Affairs (VA) Health Care System, Georgia. NMA President, 2006.
108. Nelson L. Adams, III, MD (Fig. 6.22). Undergraduate: Howard University. Medical school: Meharry Medical College. Additional: Master of Arts, New Orleans Baptist Theological Seminary. Specialty: Obstetrics/gynecology. Chief of Staff and Chair, Department of Obstetrics/Gynecology, Jackson North Medical Center, Miami, FL. Chair, Sunshine State Health Plan. NMA President, 2007.
109. Carolyn Barley Britton, MD, MS, (Fig. 6.23). Undergraduate: Oberlin College, Oberlin, OH. Medical school: New York University. Specialty: Neurology. Associate Attending Physician, Columbia University Vagelos College of Physicians and Surgeons and New York Presbyterian Milstein Hospital. Associate Professor of Neurology, Columbia University Vagelos College of

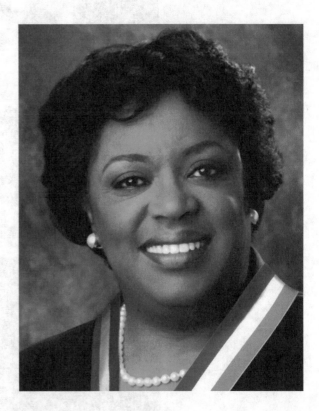

Fig. 6.20 Sandra
L. Gadson,
MD. (Photograph courtesy
of the National Medical
Association)

Fig. 6.21 Albert
W. Morris Jr.,
MD. (Photograph courtesy
of Dr. Morris)

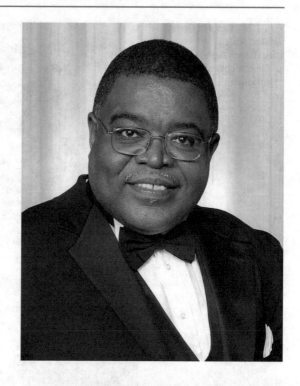

Fig. 6.22 Nelson
L. Adams, III,
MD. (Photograph courtesy
of Dr. Adams)

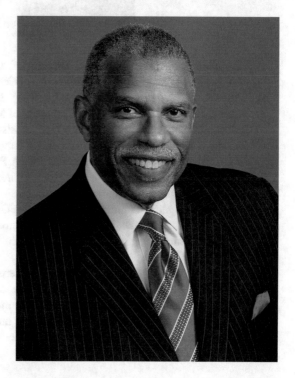

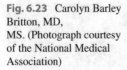

Fig. 6.23 Carolyn Barley Britton, MD, MS. (Photograph courtesy of the National Medical Association)

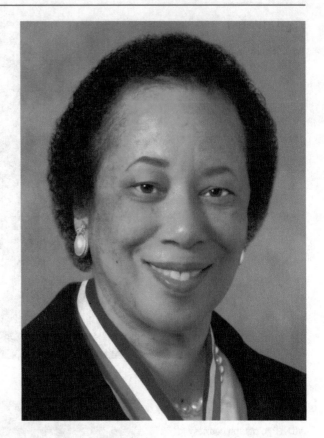

Physicians and Surgeons. Former Director of Ambulatory Care, Department of Neurology, Columbia University Medical Center. NMA President, 2008.

110. Willarda V. Edwards, MD, MBA (Fig. 6.24). Undergraduate: University of Texas at El Paso. Medical school: University of Maryland School of Medicine, Baltimore. Specialty: Internal medicine. Assistant Professor, University of Maryland Medical Center. Commander, US Navy. Member Board of Trustees, AMA. Private practice, Baltimore, MD. NMA President, 2009.

111. Leonard Weather, Jr., MD, RPh (Fig. 6.25). Undergraduate: Howard University School of Pharmacy. Medical school: Rush Medical College, Chicago, IL. Postgraduate: Training in Obstetrics/Gynecology, Johns Hopkins University Hospital, Baltimore, MD. Director, Omni Fertility and Laser Institute. Grand President, Chi Delta Mu Medical Fraternity. NMA President, 2010.

112. Cedric M. Bright, MD (Fig. 6.26). Undergraduate: Brown University, Providence, RI. Medical school: University of North Carolina School of Medicine, Chapel Hill. Specialty: Internal medicine. Associate Dean for Admissions, Professor of Internal Medicine, and Interim Associate Dean of Diversity and Inclusion, Brody School of Medicine, Greeneville NC. NMA President, 2011.

Fig. 6.24 Willarda
V. Edwards, MD,
MBA. (Photograph
courtesy of Dr. Edwards)

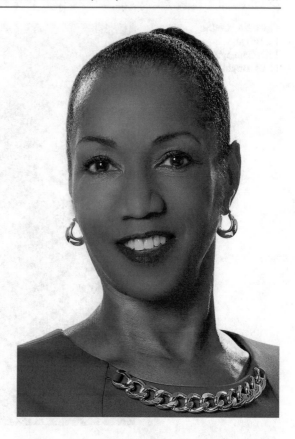

Fig. 6.25 Leonard
Weather, Jr., MD, RPh.
(Photograph courtesy of
Dr. Weather)

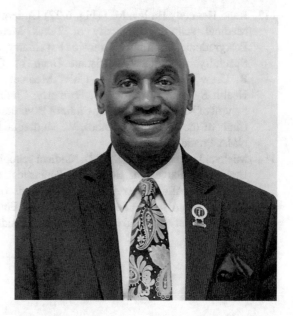

Fig. 6.26 Cedric
M. Bright,
MD. (Photograph courtesy
of Dr. Bright)

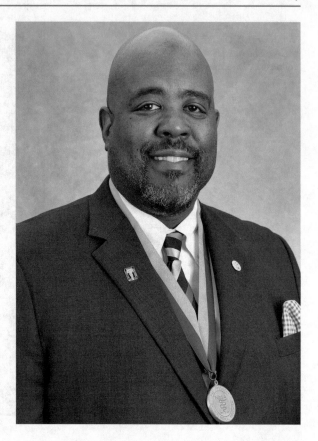

113. Rahn Kennedy Bailey, MD (Fig. 6.27) Undergraduate: Morehouse College.
Medical school: University of Texas Medical Branch at Galveston.
Postgraduate training: Forensic Psychiatry, Yale School of Medicine.
Specialty: Psychiatry. Assistant Dean of Clinical Education, Charles
R. Drew University/UCLA. Chief Medical Officer, Kedren Community
Health System, Los Angeles. Formerly, Chair of Psychiatry, Wake Forest
School of Medicine; formerly Chair of Psychiatry, Meharry Medical College.
Chair of the Board of Trustees, W. Montague Cobb/NMA Health Institute.
NMA President, 2012.
114. Michael Lenoir, MD (Fig. 6.28). Medical school: University of Texas Medical
Branch at Galveston. Specialty: Pediatrics, allergy immunity. Formerly,
Director of Allergy Services at San Francisco General Hospital. Associate
Clinical Professor in Pediatrics, UC San Francisco. CEO, Ethnic Health
American Network, Oakland, CA. NMA President, 2013.

Fig. 6.27 Rahn Kennedy Bailey, MD. (Photograph courtesy of Dr. Bailey)

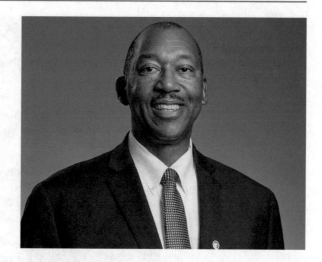

Fig. 6.28 Michael Lenoir, MD. (Photograph courtesy of Dr. Lenoir)

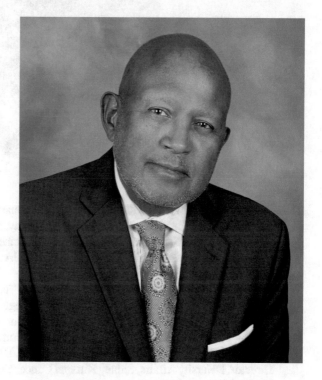

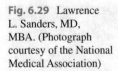

Fig. 6.29 Lawrence
L. Sanders, MD,
MBA. (Photograph
courtesy of the National
Medical Association)

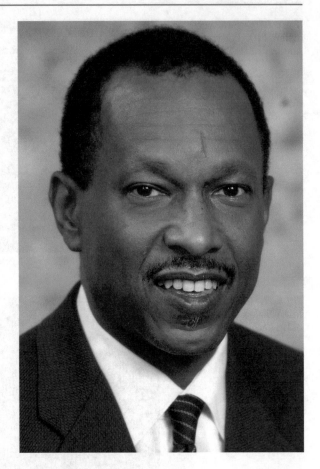

115. Lawrence L. Sanders, MD, MBA. Undergraduate: Clemson University, Clemson, SC. Medical school: Vanderbilt University, Nashville, TN. Specialty: Internal medicine. Associate Professor of Medicine, Morehouse School of Medicine, Grady Memorial Hospital, Atlanta GA. NMA President, 2014 (Fig. 6.29).
116. Edith P. Mitchell, MD (Fig. 6.30) Undergraduate: Tennessee State University, Nashville, TN. Medical school: Medical College of Virginia. Specialty: Medical oncology. Clinical Professor of Medicine and Medical Oncology, Sidney Kimmel Medical College at Thomas Jefferson Medical College, Philadelphia, PA. Director, Center to Eliminate Disparities, and Associate Director, Diversity Affairs, Sidney Kimmel Cancer Center at Thomas Jefferson Medical College. NMA President, 2015.
117. Richard Allen Williams, MD (Fig. 6.31). Undergraduate: Harvard University, graduated cum laude. Medical school: State University of New York (SUNY) Downstate Medical Center. Residencies: UC San Francisco Medical Center

Fig. 6.30 Edith
P. Mitchell,
MD. (Photograph courtesy
of Dr. Mitchell)

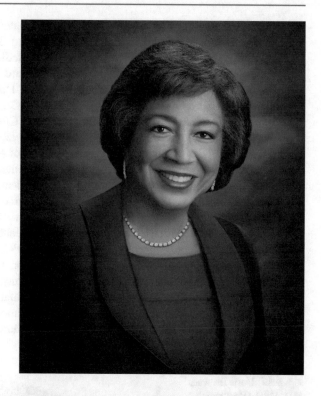

Fig. 6.31 Richard Allen
Williams,
MD. (Photograph courtesy
of Dr. Williams)

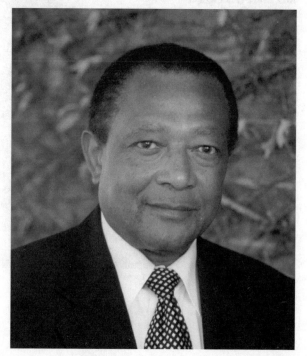

and LA County/USC Medical Center. Postgraduate: Brigham and Women's Hospital and Harvard Medical School; Oxford Round Table, England. Specialty: Cardiology. Clinical Professor of Medicine, UCLA School of Medicine. Former Instructor in Medicine, Harvard Medical School; Junior Associate in Medicine, Brigham and Women's Hospital. Former Head of Cardiology, West Los Angeles VA/UCLA Medical Center. Founder, Association of Black Cardiologists. Founder, President, and CEO, The Minority Health Institute. Author, *Textbook of Black-Related Diseases*, the first medical book by a black physician accepted into National Museum of African American History and Culture (Smithsonian Institution), and eight other books including *Blacks in Medicine* (Springer Nature, 2020). NMA President, 2016.

118. Doris Browne, MD, MPH (Fig. 6.32). Undergraduate: Tougaloo College, Tougaloo, MS. Medical school: Georgetown University, Washington, DC. Postgraduate: MPH, UCLA School of Public Health (Community Medicine). Specialty: Hematology/oncology. President and CEO, Browne and Associates, LLC. Formerly, Senior Scientific Program Director, National Cancer Institute; Deputy Medical Research and Development, US Army. NMA President, 2017.

119. Niva Lubin-Johnson, MD (Fig. 6.33). Undergraduate: Creighton University, Omaha, NE. Medical school: Southern Illinois School of Medicine. Specialty: Internal medicine. Senior Attending Physician, Mercy Hospital and Medical

Fig. 6.32 Doris Browne, MD, MPH. (Photograph courtesy of Dr. Browne)

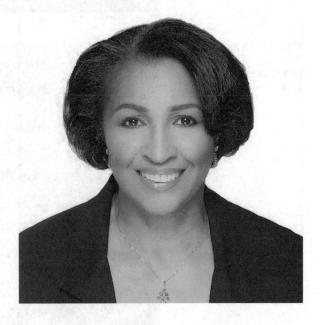

Fig. 6.33 Niva Lubin-Johnson, MD. (Photograph courtesy of Dr. Lubin-Johnson)

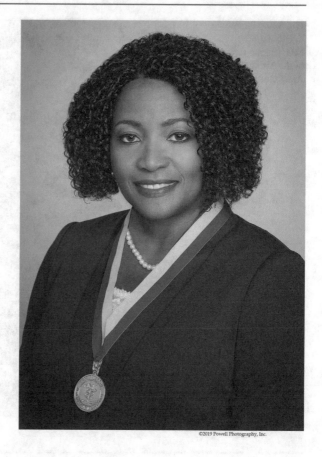

©2019 Powell Photography, Inc.

Center, Chicago IL. Clinical Instructor, University of Illinois. NMA President, 2018.

120. Oliver T. Brooks, MD (Fig. 6.34). Undergraduate: Morehouse College. Medical school: Howard University College of Medicine. Specialty: Pediatrics and adolescent medicine. Medical Director, Pediatric and Adolescent Medicine, Watts Healthcare Corporation, Los Angeles. Medical Director, Jordan and Locke High School Wellness Centers. Medical Director, LA Care Health Plan. Vice-Chair of the Obstetrics/Pediatrics Department, Martin Luther King, Jr. Community Hospital in South Los Angeles. NMA President, 2019.

Fig. 6.34 Oliver
T. Brooks,
MD. (Photograph courtesy
of the National Medical
Association)

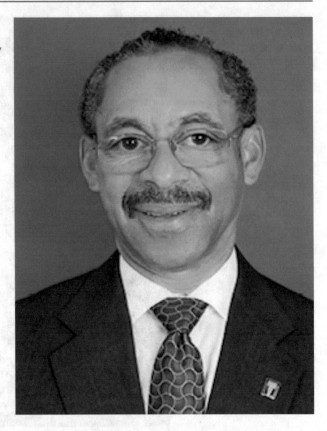

Additional Members of the Honor Roll of Distinguished African American Physicians and Other Healthcare Professionals

1. Joycelyn Elders, MD, MS (Fig. 6.35). 15th US Surgeon General. First African American and the second woman to head the US Public Health Service. First person to be board certified in pediatric endocrinology in the state of Arkansas. Growing up on a farm in rural poverty, she worked the fields while attending segregated schools. Earned a scholarship to the black liberal arts Philander Smith College, Little Rock, scrubbing floors to pay tuition. Joined the US Army, trained in physical therapy at the Brooke Army Medical Center at Fort Sam Houston, Texas. Enrolled at the University of Arkansas Medical School, Little Rock, on the GI Bill. Internship in pediatrics at the University of Minnesota; residency at University of Arkansas; chief resident in charge of the all-white, all-male residents and interns. Earned an MS in biochemistry and became assistant professor of pediatrics in 1971 and full professor in 1976. Governor William Clinton appointed her head of the Arkansas Department of Health in 1987 and, when he gained the presidency, appointed

Fig. 6.35 M. Joycelyn Elders, MD. (Photograph courtesy of the National Institutes of Health)

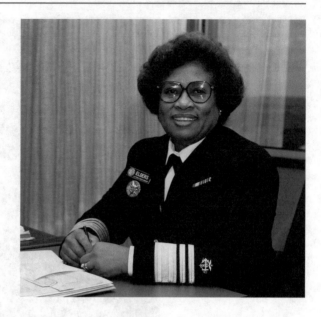

her US Surgeon General in 1993. Returned to the University of Arkansas as a faculty researcher and professor of pediatric endocrinology. Autobiography: *Joycelyn Elders, MD: From Sharecropper's Daughter to Surgeon General of the United States of America* (1996). Now professor emeritus at the University of Arkansas School of Medicine, she remains active in public health education [7].

2. David Satcher, MD, PhD (Fig. 6.36). 16th US Surgeon General. Undergraduate: Morehouse College. Medical school and postgraduate (PhD, Cytogenetics): Case Western Reserve University, Cleveland, OH. Administrative and faculty positions at the Charles R. Drew Postgraduate Medical School, the King-Drew Sickle Cell Center, and UCLA's School of Public Health, Los Angeles, CA. Former Chair of the Department of Community Medicine and Family Practice at Charles R. Drew University of Medicine and Science and served as President of Drew University, Meharry Medical College, and Morehouse School of Medicine, the only African American physician to serve as president of three medical schools in succession. Appointed director of the Centers for Disease Control and Prevention (CDC) in 1993. Appointed by President Clinton as US Surgeon General in 1998, served concurrently as Assistant Secretary for Health, US Department of Health and Human Services. Currently, Founding Director and Senior Advisor, Satcher Health Leadership Institute, Department of Community Health and Preventive Medicine, Morehouse School of Medicine [8].

3. Regina Benjamin, MD, MBA (Fig. 6.37). 18th US Surgeon General. Undergraduate: Xavier University, New Orleans, LA; Medical school: University of Alabama, Birmingham. Postgraduate: MBA, Tulane University, New Orleans, LA. Served as Associate Dean for Rural Health at the University

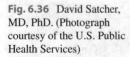

Fig. 6.36 David Satcher, MD, PhD. (Photograph courtesy of the U.S. Public Health Services)

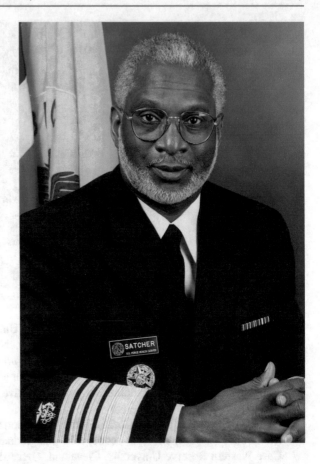

of South Alabama and Director of the Alabama Area Health Education Center, which provides educational opportunities and mentoring to area medical students. Appointed US Surgeon General by President Barack Obama in 2009. Founder and CEO of the rural BayouClinic in Bayou La Batre, LA, serving the underserved in a small fishing village on the Gulf Coast of Alabama, where 80% of the citizens live below the poverty level. Currently occupies an endowed chair in health sciences at her alma mater, Xavier University. Founder of Gulf States Health Policy Center in Bayou La Batre, working to improve health outcomes in the Gulf States [9].

4. Vice Admiral Jerome M. Adams, MD, MPH (Fig. 6.38). 20th US Surgeon General, Medical school: Indiana University School of Medicine, Indianapolis, IN. Postgraduate: MPH (Chronic Disease Prevention), UC Berkeley. Specialty: Anesthesiology. Holds the rank of Vice Admiral in the US Public Health Service. Indiana Health Commissioner and faculty member of Indiana University. Appointed US Surgeon General by President Donald Trump in 2017. Recognized as a leading expert in the substance abuse crisis, and has pledged to combat the opioid crisis confronting the nation [10]. Has taken a leading role in combating the coronavirus crisis facing the United States.

Fig. 6.37 Regina Benjamin, MD, MBA. (Photograph courtesy of the Department of Health and Human Services)

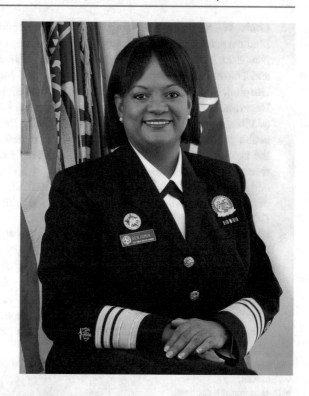

Fig. 6.38 Vice Admiral Jerome M. Adams, MD, MPH. (Courtesy U.S. Public Health Service)

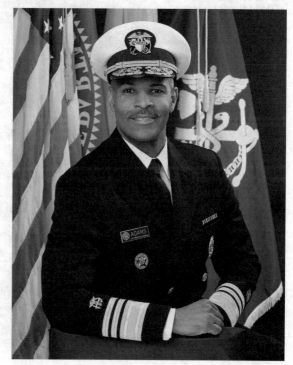

5. Louis W. Sullivan, MD (Fig. 6.39). Undergraduate: Morehouse College. Medical school: Boston University School of Medicine. Postgraduate training: New York Hospital—Cornell Medical Center, Massachusetts General Hospital, and Thorndike Memorial Laboratory of Harvard Medical School, Boston City Hospital. Specialties: Internal medicine and hematology. As secretary of the US Department of Health and Human Services in the President George H.W. Bush administration (1989–1993), launched Healthy People 2000 (a blueprint for health promotion/disease prevention), campaigned against tobacco, promoted the use of seat belts in vehicles, and improved FDA food labels. Prominent researcher in hematology at Boston University and at Harvard. Founding Dean and President of the Morehouse School of Medicine. Currently, Chair and CEO of the Sullivan Alliance to Transform the Health Professions, Washington, DC [11].

6. Claude H. Organ, MD (1926–2005) (Fig. 6.40). Undergraduate: Xavier University. Medical school: Creighton University School of Medicine. General surgeon, educator, and author (*A Century of Black Surgeons: The USA Experience*). First African American to head the surgical department at Creighton (Professor and Chair, 1971). Later also Professor at the University of Oklahoma and at UC Davis. A founder of the Society of Black Academic Surgeons. The second black president of the American College of Surgeons.

Fig. 6.39 Louis W. Sullivan, MD. (Photograph courtesy of the National Library of Medicine)

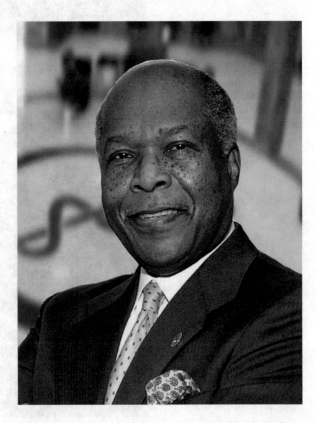

Fig. 6.40 Claude
H. Organ,
MD. (Photograph courtesy
of the Organ family)

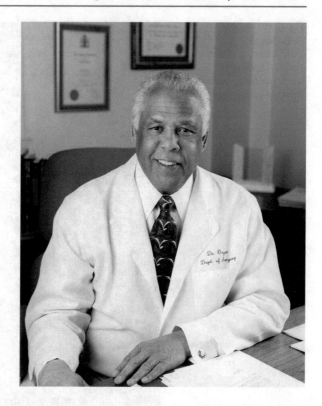

Member of the editorial board of JAMA and the first African American editor
of the *Archives of Surgery*. Only male to receive the Nina Starr Braunwald
Award (1993) from the Association of Women Surgeons for "outstanding service to the advancement of women in surgery."

7. Lasalle D. Leffall, Jr., MD (1930–2019) (Fig. 6.41). Undergraduate: BS (*summa
cum laude*) Florida A&M University, Tallahassee. Medical school: Howard
University College of Medicine. Fellowship: Surgical oncology, Memorial
Sloan Kettering Cancer Center, New York City, remaining there before serving
in the US Army Medical Corps (Chief of General Surgery, US Army Hospital
in Munich, Germany, 1960–1961). Late distinguished Charles R. Drew
Professor and Chair of the Department of Surgery at Howard University College
of Medicine. The first African American to be President of the American
College of Surgeons and of the American Cancer Society. First African
American to be President of the following professional societies: American
Cancer Society, where he focused needed attention on the disparities in cancer
incidence, diagnosis, treatment, and mortality among African Americans;
Society of Surgical Oncology; and the American College of Surgery. Member
of Alpha Omega Alpha Honor Medical Society. Awarded Howard's prestigious
Faculty Award, their highest academic honor, over 30 times, which is unprece-
dented in the university's 150-year history. Published memories: *No Boundaries:
A Cancer Surgeon's Odyssey* (2005).

Fig. 6.41 Lasalle
D. Leffall, Jr.,
MD. (Courtesy of the
National Library of
Medicine, with permission
from the Leffall family)

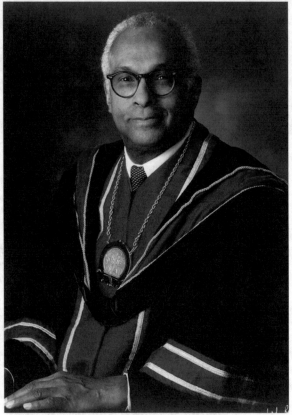

Courtesy LaSalle D. Leffall, Jr., M.D.

8. Keith L. Black, MD (Fig. 6.42). College and medical school: University of Michigan. Specialty: Neurosurgery. Former Head of the UCLA Comprehensive Brain Tumor Program. Currently Chair of Neurosurgery and Director of the Maxine Dunitz Neurosurgical Institute at Cedars Sinai Medical Center in Los Angeles. Research focuses on biology of blood-brain barrier and biochemical modulation of the blood-brain tumor barrier, targeted drug delivery, tumor immunology, cancer vaccines, cancer stem cells, microwave tumor ablation, nanotechnology for drug delivery, optical guided surgery for brain tumors, and Alzheimer's retinal imaging.

9. Ludlow B. Creary, MD, MPH (Fig. 6.43). Undergraduate: Long Island University, Brooklyn, NY. Medical school: Howard University College of Medicine. Postgraduate: MPH, Fielding School of Public Health at UCLA. Professor and inaugural Chair, Department of Family Medicine, Charles R. Drew University of Medicine and Science/UCLA for more than two decades. One of the founders of the Dr. Martin Luther King, Jr. Community Hospital in Watts. Distinguished Service Award from the National Medical Association and the Legacy Award from National Medical Fellowships. Inducted into the Hall of Fame at the Fielding School of Public Health at UCLA in 2019. President of the philanthropic Creary Family Foundation.

Fig. 6.42 Keith L. Black, MD. (Photograph ©The Beverly Hills Photographer, courtesy of Kareem Assassa)

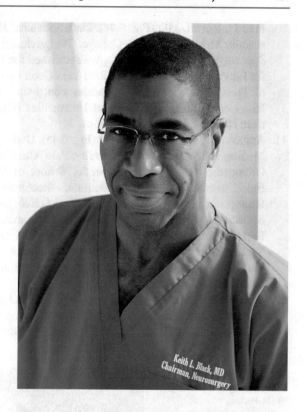

Fig. 6.43 Ludlow B. Creary, MD, MPH. (Photograph courtesy of Dr. Creary)

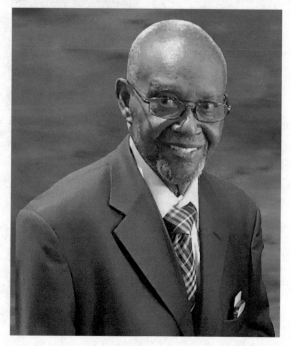

10. Fred D. Parrott, MD (Fig. 6.44). Undergraduate: Howard University. Medical school: Meharry Medical College. Postgraduate: University of Minnesota. Specialty: Obstetrics/gynecology. Established the Real Men Cook Foundation for Education in 1984 and the Real Men Cook Foundation for Early Detection of Prostate Cancer in 1994. Major contributor to the medical schools of Historically Black Colleges and Universities (HBCU). 2020 Legacy Award from National Medical Fellowships.
11. Augustus A. White III, MD, PhD (Fig. 6.45). Undergraduate: Brown University. Medical school: Stanford University, Palo Alto CA. Postgraduate: Residency, Orthopedic surgery, Yale University School of Medicine; PhD, Orthopedic Biomechanics, Karolinska Institute, Stockholm, Sweden. Professor of Orthopedic Surgery at Harvard Medical School for 41 years. Notable for his contributions to the delivery of equitable humane healthcare. Received the Bronze Star for his service as a military surgeon in Vietnam and the Distinguished Service Award from the NMA. Currently the Ellen and Melvin Gordon Distinguished Professor of Medical Education and Professor of Surgery at Harvard Medical School.
12. Charles H. Epps, Jr., MD (Fig. 6.46). Medical school: Howard University College of Medicine. Specialty: Orthopedic surgery with a focus on children with insufficient limbs. Taught thousands of students and residents. Former

Fig. 6.44 Fred D. Parrott, MD. (Photograph courtesy of Dr. Parrott)

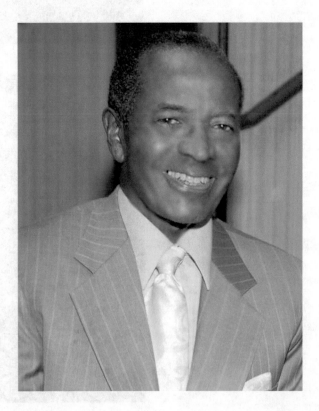

Fig. 6.45 Augustus
A. White III, MD,
PhD. (Photograph courtesy
of Dr. White)

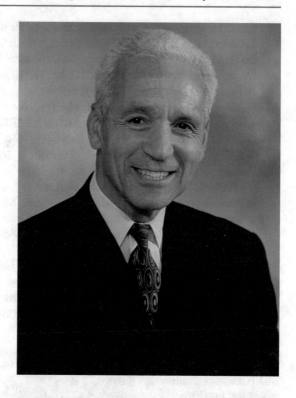

Fig. 6.46 Charles
H. Epps, Jr.,
MD. (Photograph courtesy
of daughter Roselyn
E. Epps, MD)

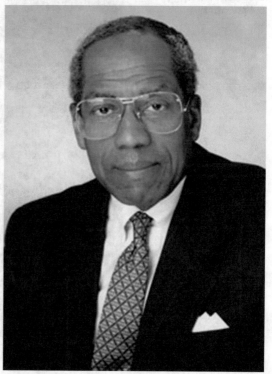

Chair of Orthopedics and former Dean at Howard. First African American President of the American Orthopaedic Association. Publications: Senior editor, *African-American Medical Pioneers* (1994); editor, *Complications in Orthopaedic Surgery*, Vols I and II (1986/1994); and co-editor of *Complications in Pediatric Orthopaedic Surgery*, (1994).

13. Roselyn Payne Epps, MD, MPH, MA (Fig. 6.47). Undergraduate and medical school: Howard University. Postgraduate: MPH, Johns Hopkins University, Baltimore, MD; MA Interdisciplinary Studies, American University, Washington, DC. Specialties: Pediatrics and public health. Former Commissioner of Public Health for Washington, DC. First African American woman President of the American Academy of Pediatrics in DC and first African woman President of the American Medical Women's Association. Under the auspices of the American Medical Women's Association, senior editor of *The Women's Complete Healthbook* (1995), one of the first manuals of its kind.

14. Wayne J. Riley, MD, MPH, MBA (Fig. 6.48). Undergraduate: Yale University. Medical school: Morehouse School of Medicine. Postgraduate: MPH, Tulane University School of Public Health and Tropical Medicine; MBA, Rice University, Houston, TX. Residency: Baylor College of Medicine. Specialty:

Fig. 6.47 Roselyn Payne Epps, MD, MPH, MD. (Photograph courtesy of daughter Roselyn E. Epps, MD)

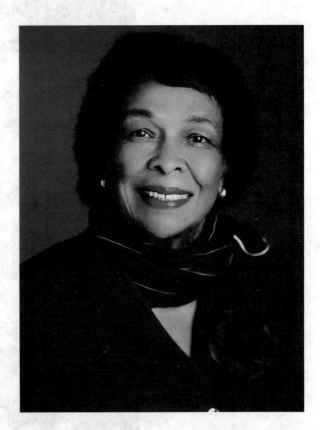

Fig. 6.48 Wayne J. Riley, MD, MPH, MBA. (Photograph courtesy of Dr. Riley)

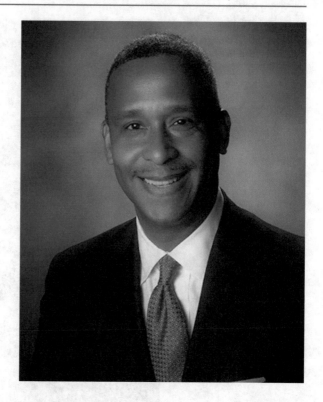

Internal medicine. President Emeritus, American College of Physicians. Member, National Academy of Medicine. Former Chair, Section on the Administration of Health Services, Education, and Research, National Academy of Medicine. Former President, Meharry Medical College. Fellow and Member, Board of Trustees, New York Academy of Medicine; Secretary and Member, Board of Trustees, Arnold P. Gold Foundation. Currently, President, SUNY Downstate Health Sciences University, and Professor of Internal Medicine and Health Policy and Management at SUNY.

15. Lonnie R. Bristow, MD (Fig. 6.49). Undergraduate: Morehouse College and City College of New York. Medical school: New York University. Specialties: Internal medicine, occupational medicine. First African American elected President of the American Medical Association (AMA) (1995–1996). During tenure as Chair of the AMA Board of Trustees, successful in obtaining AMA support for the federal government's plan for healthcare reform put forth by the Clinton Administration. Currently an active member of the National Academy of Medicine, one of three academies that make up the National Academies of Sciences, Engineering, and Medicine in the United States. Received the 2009 NYU Health Science Award. Has articulated a core set of principles regarding patients that he feels every physician is obligated to observe: compassion, competence, courtesy, and honesty.

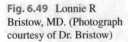
Fig. 6.49 Lonnie R
Bristow, MD. (Photograph
courtesy of Dr. Bristow)

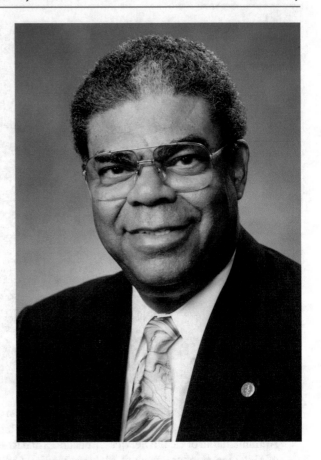

16. Patrice A. Harris, MD, MA (Fig. 6.50). Undergraduate, medical school, post-graduate: West Virginia University, Morgantown, WV. Residency and fellow-ships: Child, adolescent, and forensic psychiatry, Emory University School of Medicine. Forensic and child/adolescent psychiatrist from Cartersville, GA. Served as Chief Health Officer for Fulton County, GA, where she advanced a program to integrate public and behavioral health and primary care. Adjunct assistant clinical professor at the Morehouse School of Medicine, as well as an adjunct assistant professor in the Emory Department of Psychiatry and Behavioral Sciences. In June 2019, sworn in as the first black woman to lead the AMA. Prior to becoming AMA President, she was a member of the Board of Directors from 2011 and Chair from 2016. Chair of the AMA's Opioid Task Force.
17. Clyde W. Yancy, MD, MSc (Fig. 6.51). Medical school: Tulane University School of Medicine. Vice Dean, Diversity and Inclusion; Magerstadt Endowed Professor of Medicine; Professor of Medical Social Sciences; and Chief of Cardiology at Northwestern University, Feinberg School of Medicine, Evanston, IL. President of the American Heart Association (2009–2010). Author of "The Role of Race in Heart Failure Therapy" (*Current Cardiology Reports*, 2002).

Fig. 6.50 Patrice
A. Harris, MD,
MA. (Photograph courtesy
of Dr. Harris)

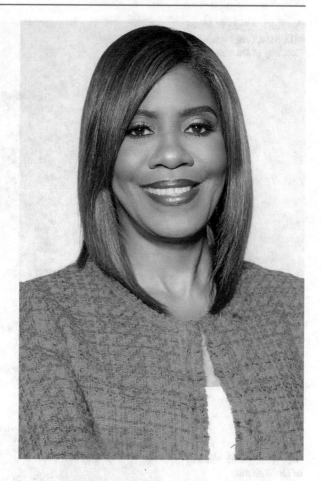

Deputy Editor, *JAMA Cardiology*; and serves on the editorial boards for *Journal of the American College of Cardiology, Circulation, American Heart Journal,* and *JACC Heart Failure.* As a revered and legendary educator and researcher in heart failure, received the Dr. Daniel D. Savage Science Award from the ABC.

18. Kim A. Williams, MD (Fig. 6.52). Undergraduate: University of Chicago. Medical School: University of Chicago Pritzker School of Medicine. Residency and fellowship: Emory University Hospital and the University of Chicago Medical Center. James B. Herrick Professor of Medicine and Chief of the Division of Cardiology at Rush University in Chicago, specializing in prevention and imaging. Has served on numerous national committees and boards, including President of the American College of Cardiology, President of the American Society of Nuclear Cardiology, and Chair of the Board of Directors of the ABC. Founder of the Urban Cardiology Initiative in Detroit, Michigan, to reduce ethnic heart care disparities; continues community-based efforts in Chicago at Rush. Among the world's leaders in cardiac imaging, he received the Dr. Daniel D. Savage Science Award from the ABC.

Fig. 6.51 Clyde W. Yancy, MD, MSc. (Photograph Courtesy of Dr. Yancy)

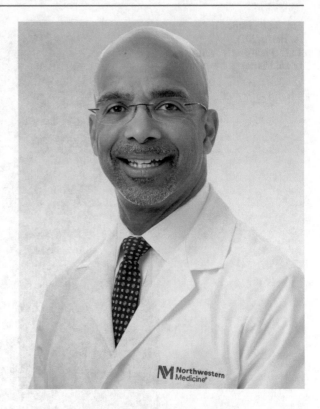

Fig. 6.52 Kim A. Williams, MD. (Photograph courtesy of Dr. Williams)

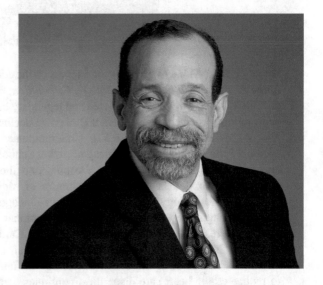

19. James E. K. Hildreth, PhD, MD (Fig. 6.53). Undergraduate: BS Chemistry (*magna* cum *laude*) from Harvard University, selected as the first African American Rhodes Scholar from Arkansas. Postgraduate: PhD in Immunology, University of Oxford, Oxford, UK. Medical school: Johns Hopkins School of Medicine where he later became the first African American Full Professor in the basic sciences. A distinguished medical researcher, especially in the fight against HIV/AIDS, he was elected to Institute of Medicine (now known as the National Academy of Medicine, one of three academies that make up the US National Academies of Sciences, Engineering, and Medicine). Former Dean of the College of Biological Sciences at UC Davis and professor in the Departments of Molecular Biology and Internal Medicine at the UC Davis School of Medicine. Currently serves as the 12th President and Chief Executive Officer of Meharry Medical College

20. David M. Carlisle, MD, PhD (Fig. 6.54). Undergraduate: Wesleyan University, Middletown, CT. Medical school: Brown University. Postgraduate: MPH and PhD, Health Services, UCLA Fielding School of Public Health. Robert Wood

Fig. 6.53 James E. K. Hildreth, PhD, MD. (Photograph courtesy of Dr. Hildreth)

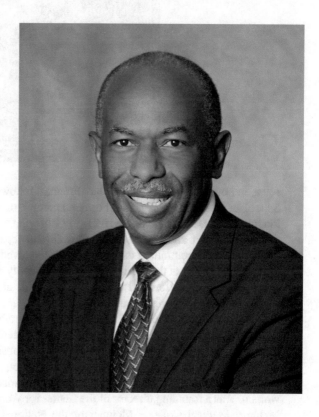

Fig. 6.54 David
M. Carlisle, MD,
PhD. (Photograph courtesy
of Dr. Carlisle)

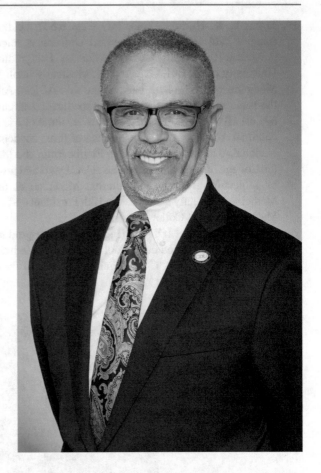

Johnson Foundation Clinical Scholars Program fellowship at the David Geffen
School of Medicine at UCLA. Former Director of the Office of Statewide
Planning and Development (OSHPD) in California, overseeing its first health
disparities report and increased scholarship and repayment opportunities for
health providers committed to practice in underserved communities. Currently
President and CEO of the Charles R. Drew University of Medicine and Science/
UCLA in Watts, California. Professor of Medicine at Drew University and an
Adjunct Professor of Medicine at UCLA.

21. Valerie Montgomery Rice, MD (Fig. 6.55). Undergraduate: Georgia Institute of
Technology, Atlanta. Medical school: Harvard Medical School. Residency:
Emory University School of Medicine. Expert in obstetrics/gynecology and a
distinguished researcher in infertility, focusing on the health problems of
women of color, particularly on disproportionate maternal mortality in black
women. Was a founding director of the Center for Women's Health Research at
Meharry Medical College. Member of the National Academy of Medicine.
Currently President and Dean, Morehouse School of Medicine.

Fig. 6.55 Valerie Montgomery Rice, MD. (Photograph courtesy of Dr. Rice)

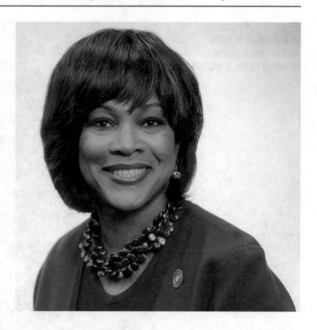

22. Wayne A.I. Frederick, MD, MBA (Fig. 6.56). Undergraduate and medical school: Bachelor of Science (BS)/MD dual degree program, Howard University. Postgraduate: Research and fellowship in surgical oncology, University of Texas MD Anderson Cancer Center. Born in Trinidad, he entered Howard at age 16 fueled by his desire to become a physician and to learn more about sickle cell anemia. A consummate teacher, researcher, and exponent of equity and of the recognition of unconscious bias in medicine. Medical research focuses on narrowing racial, ethnic, and gender disparities in cancer care outcomes, especially concerning gastrointestinal disease. He writes and lectures on the impact of HBCUs and the underrepresentation of African American men in medical school. Currently President of Howard University College of Medicine, having served previously as Provost and Chief Academic Officer.

23. Harold P. Freeman, MD (Fig. 6.57). Undergraduate: Catholic University of America, Washington, DC. Medical school: Howard University College of Medicine. Founder, President, and CEO of the Harold P. Freeman Patient Navigation Institute in New York City. Pioneered the concept of "patient navigation," to provide low-income patients with personal guides through the healthcare system. Director of Surgery at Harlem Hospital (1974—99); Professor of Clinical Surgery at Columbia University College of Physicians and Surgeons. Founder, Past President, and Chair Emeritus of the Ralph Lauren Center for Cancer Care and Prevention. Founding Director of the National Cancer Institute (NCI) Center to Reduce Cancer Health Disparities (2001–2005) while also serving as Associate Director of the NCI. Founder and Medical Director of the Breast Examination Center of Harlem (a program of Memorial Sloan Kettering Cancer Center), since 1979. Elected to the Institute of Medicine

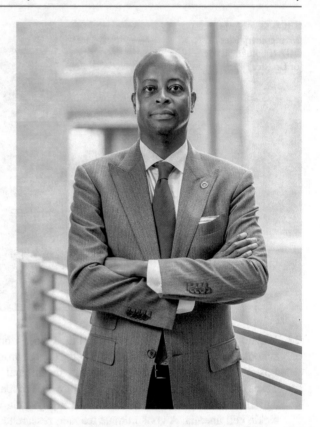

Fig. 6.56 Wayne
A.I. Frederick, MD,
MBA. (Photograph
courtesy of Dr. Frederick)

(now known as the National Academy of Medicine) in 1997. National President of the American Cancer Society (1988–1989); chief architect of the American Cancer Society initiative on *Cancer in the Poor*, for which the Harold P. Freeman Award was established in 1990 to honor his work in that field. Leading authority on the interrelationships between race, poverty, and cancer, awarded the 2000 Mary Woodard Lasker Public Service Award for addressing the social determinants of disease.

24. Cato T. Laurencin, MD, PhD (Fig. 6.58). Undergraduate: BSE chemical engineering, Princeton University, Princeton, NJ. Medical school: Harvard Medical School (*magna* cum *laude*). Postgraduate: PhD, Biochemical Engineering/ Biotechnology, Massachusetts Institute of Technology, Cambridge, MA. Albert and Wilda Van Dusen distinguished endowed Professor of Orthopedic Surgery, the eighth designated university professor in the university's 135-year history. Professor of Chemical, Materials, and Biomedical Engineering and CEO of the Connecticut Convergence Institute for Translation in Regenerative Engineering at the University of Connecticut, formerly serving there as Dean of the Medical School and Vice President for Health Affairs. Received NIH Director's Pioneer Award for work in regenerative engineering and the Philip Hauge Abelson Prize from the American Association for the Advancement of Science (AAAS).

Fig. 6.57 Harold
P. Freeman
MD. (Photograph courtesy
of Dr. Freeman)

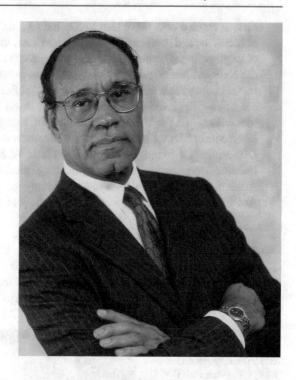

Fig. 6.58 Cato
T. Laurencin, MD,
PhD. (Photograph courtesy
of Dr. Laurencin)

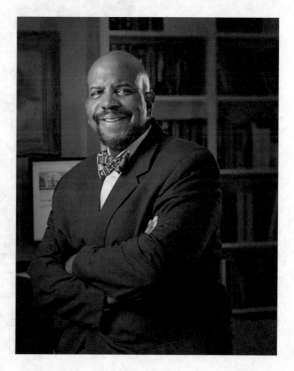

First to receive both the Walsh McDermott Medal from the National Academy of Medicine and the Simon Ramo Founder's Award from the National Academy of Engineering. The first orthopedic surgeon and first black physician to receive the National Medal of Technology and Innovation, the nation's highest honor for technological achievement, from President Barack Obama in a White House ceremony. Received the AAAS Mentor Award, the Beckman Award for Mentoring, and the Presidential Award for Excellence in Science, Math, and Engineering Mentoring. Editor in Chief, *Journal of Racial and Ethnic Health Disparities*. Co-founder and Founding Chair, W. Montague Cobb/NMA Health Institute, dedicated to addressing health disparities. Member of the National Academy of Medicine, National Academy of Engineering, and American Academy of Arts and Sciences; elected fellow of a number of international science academies.

25. W. Michael Byrd, MD, MPH (Fig. 6.59). Undergraduate: Morehouse College. Medical school: Meharry Medical College. Postgraduate: MPH, Harvard H. T. Chan School of Public Health, where he has taught for over 25 years as a senior research scientist in the Department of Health Policy and Management. Battalion Surgeon in the US Army Medical Corps on active duty in the Vietnam

Fig. 6.59 W. Michael Byrd, MD, MPH. (Photograph ©Don West, with permission)

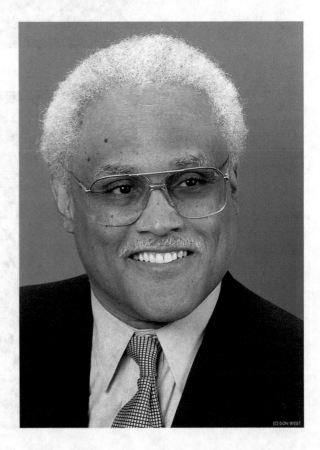

War, awarded the Bronze Star Medal. Obstetrician and gynecologist who has practiced his specialty for over four decades. A nationally and internationally recognized authority on African American and disadvantaged population health and healthcare; racial and ethnic disparities; health reform; health equity; and health policy and health service delivery, called upon as a consultant by presidential administrations, the National Academy of Medicine, the Congressional Black Caucus, the NAACP, and the NMA. Author of the book *An American Health Dilemma:* (Vol. 1) *A Medical History of African Americans and the Problem of Race: Beginnings to 1900* and (Vol. 2) *Race, Medicine, and Health Care in the United States, 1900–2000*, written with his wife and colleague Dr. Linda A. Clayton. The authors are currently working on the 2nd edition and 3rd volume.

26. Linda A. Clayton, MD, MPH (Fig. 6.60). Undergraduate: North Carolina Central University, Durham. Medical school: Duke University Medical School, Durham, NC. Postgraduate: MPH, Harvard H. T. Chan School of Public Health. Obstetrician and gynecologist and the first African American woman to be subspecialty trained in surgical gynecologic oncology. For several decades has provided direct patient care through radical pelvic surgery and other oncologic

Fig. 6.60 Linda A. Clayton, MD, MPH. (Photograph ©Don West, with permission)

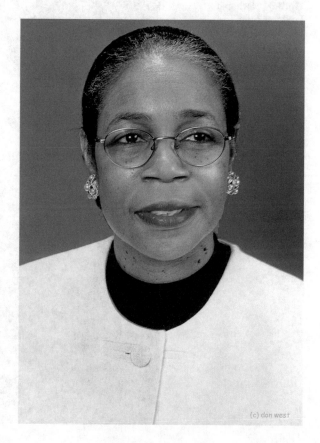

therapeutic interventions for women with pelvic malignancies. Extensive experience in enrolling patients into cancer clinical trials; has conducted biomedical research in laboratory and clinical settings since the early 1980s. Has provided expert medical and policy analysis since the 1990s. A nationally and internationally recognized authority on African American and disadvantaged population health; racial and ethnic disparities; health reform; and health equity. Called upon as a consultant by presidential administrations, the National Cancer Institute, the Congressional Black Caucus, the Office of Minority Health, and the NMA. Senior research scientist in the Department of Health Policy and Management at the Harvard H. T. Chan School of Public Health. Author of the book: *An American Health Dilemma:* (Vol. 1) *A Medical History of African Americans and the Problem of Race: Beginnings to 1900* and (Vol. 2) *Race, Medicine, and Health Care in the United States, 1900–2000*, written with her husband and colleague Dr. W. Michael Byrd; the authors are currently working on the 2nd edition and 3rd volume.

27. Deborah Prothrow-Stith, MD (Fig. 6.61). Undergraduate: Spelman College, Atlanta, GA. Medical school: Harvard Medical School. Residency: Internal

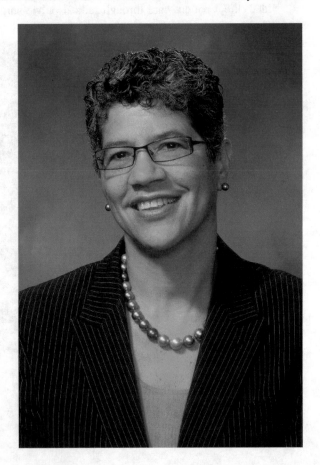

Fig. 6.61 Deborah Prothrow-Stith, MD. (Photograph courtesy of Dr. Prothrow-Stith)

medicine, Boston City Hospital. Dean and Professor of Medicine, College of Medicine at Charles R. Drew University of Medicine and Science/ UCLA. Internationally recognized public health leader, previously served as the Henry Pickering Walcott Professor of Public Health Practice and Associate Dean for Diversity at the Harvard H. T. Chan School of Public Health. Working as a physician in inner-city Boston, broke new ground in defining youth violence as a public health problem. Author of *Deadly Consequences: How Violence Is Destroying Our Teenage Population and a Plan to Begin Solving the Problem* (1991), the first book to present the public health perspective on violence; co-author *of Murder Is No Accident: Understanding and Preventing Youth Violence in America* (2004). Appointed the first woman Commissioner of Public Health for Massachusetts by Governor Michael Dukakis. Established the nation's first Office of Violence Prevention in a state department of public health, expanded prevention programs for HIV/AIDS, and increased drug treatment and rehabilitation programs. Lived in Tanzania during her husband's tenure as US Ambassador, working with Muhimbili National Hospital and an NGO that runs the first HIV clinic in Tanzania. Member of the National Academy of Medicine. Recipient of the 1993 World Health Day Award, the 1989 Secretary of Health and Human Service Award, and a Presidential appointment to the National Commission on Crime Control and Prevention.

28. Julian Haywood, MD (Fig. 6.62) Undergraduate: Hampton Institute (high honors). Medical school: Howard University, with honors. Residency: Internal Medicine, LA County General Hospital. Cardiology fellowship: White Memorial Hospital, Los Angeles. Traveling fellowship under Oxford University Regius Professor of Medicine George Pickering. Joined faculty University of Southern California in 1963. Retired in 2019 as Professor Emeritus in Medicine, USC, and Honored Clinical Professor of Medicine, Loma Linda University School of Medicine. Extensive publication in hypertension, population research, clinical cardiology and arrhythmias, heart disease in sickle cell anemia patients, and biomedical engineering. Established the coronary care unit at LA County General Hospital, one of the first in the world (1966), which was renamed for him in 2016; developed the first digital heart rhythm monitor (1969); established the Comprehensive Sickle Cell Center at LA County General Hospital, one of the first in the nation (1972); a Founding Member of ABC (1974). Member of the Alpha Omega Alpha Honor Medical Society and a Distinguished Alumnus of Hampton and Howard Universities.

Alvin F. Poussaint, MD (Fig. 6.63). Undergraduate: Columbia University. Medical school: Cornell University. Postgraduate training: UCLA Neuropsychiatric Institute, serving as Chief Resident in Psychiatry; MS, Psychopharmacology. Southern Field Director of the Medical Committee for Human Rights in Jackson, Mississippi (1965–1967), providing medical care to civil rights workers and aiding desegregation of hospitals and health facilities throughout the South. Medical foot soldier for the march from Selma to Montgomery, Alabama, in March 1965 with Rev. Dr. Martin Luther King, Jr. Joined Tufts Medical School faculty as director of a psychiatry program in a

Fig. 6.62 L. Julian Haywood, MD. (Photograph courtesy of Dr. Haywood)

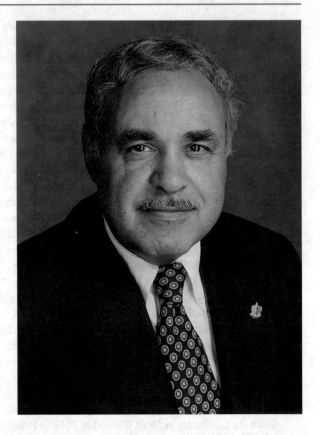

low-income housing development before joining Harvard Medical School faculty in 1969, serving as Dean of Students and Director of the Office of Recruitment and Multicultural Affairs. Instrumental in expanding the enrollment of underrepresented medical students and mentoring their academic careers. Also served on the staff of Harvard's Judge Baker's Children's Center. Currently Professor of Psychiatry, Emeritus, Harvard Medical School. Author of *Why Blacks Kill Blacks* (1972); co-author of *Raising Black Children* (1992); and co-author of *Lay My Burden Down* (2000). Awarded the Herbert W. Nickens Award, recognizing outstanding contributions promoting justice in medical education and healthcare by the Association of American Medical Colleges in 2010. Distinguished life fellow of the American Psychiatric Association, a fellow of the AAAS, a life member of the American Academy of Child and Adolescent Psychiatry, and a member of the American Academy of Arts and Sciences. Recipient of the NMA Distinguished Service Award.

29. Risa Lavizzo-Mourey, MD, MBA (Fig. 6.64) Medical school: Harvard Medical School. Internship and residency: Internal Medicine, Brigham and Women's Hospital, Boston, MA. Postgraduate: MBA, Wharton School of the University of Pennsylvania. President Emerita and former CEO, Robert Wood Johnson

Fig. 6.63 Alvin
F. Poussaint,
MD. (Photograph courtesy
of Dr. Poussaint)

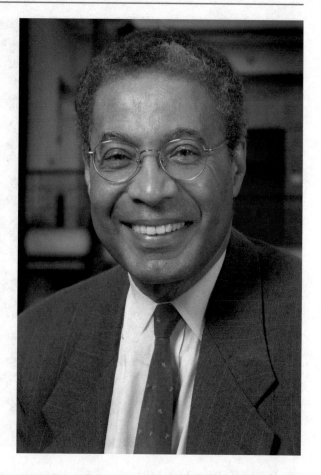

Foundation (RWJF) (2003–2017), where she administered an endowment of $10.5 billion dollars, the nation's largest charitable fund devoted entirely to health. Spearheaded bold health initiatives during her tenure such as creating healthier, more equitable communities; strengthening the integration of health systems and services; and ensuring every child in the United States has the opportunity to grow up at a healthy weight. This work culminated in the Foundation's vision of building a culture of health, enabling everyone in America to live longer, healthier lives. Served as deputy administrator for what is now the Agency for Healthcare Research and Quality (AHRQ) and has worked on the White House Health Care Reform Task Force. Served on numerous federal advisory committees and was appointed by President Barack Obama to the President's Council on Fitness, Sports, and Nutrition. Currently serves as the 19th *Penn Integrates Knowledge* University Professor at the University of Pennsylvania, with joint faculty appointments at the Perelman School of Medicine, the School of Nursing, and the Wharton School. Recipient of the Distinguished Service Award from the NMA.

Fig. 6.64 Risa Lavizzo-Mourey, MD. (Photograph courtesy of Dr. Lavizzo-Mourey)

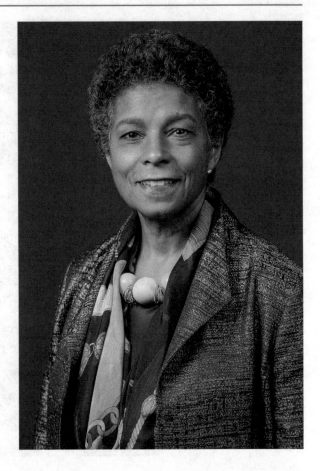

30. Robert K. Ross, MD, MPA (Fig. 6.65). Undergraduate, medical school, postgraduate (Master of Public Administration): University of Pennsylvania. Currently, President and CEO of The California Endowment, a private, statewide health foundation established in 1996 to address the health needs of Californians. Prior to his appointment in September 2000, served as director of the Health and Human Services Agency for the County of San Diego from 1993 to 2000. Extensive background in health philanthropy as a public health administrator and as a clinician. Commissioner, Philadelphia Department of Public Health; medical director for LINK School-Based Clinic Program, Camden NJ; instructor of clinical medicine, Children's Hospital of Philadelphia; and faculty member at San Diego State University's School of Public Health. Member of the President's Advisory Commission on Educational Excellence for African Americans; Co-chair, Diversity in Philanthropy Coalition; member of the California Health Benefit Exchange Board, the Rockefeller Philanthropy Advisors Board, National Vaccine Advisory Committee, and on the boards of Grantmakers in Health, the National Marrow Donor Program, San Diego United Way, and the Jackie Robinson YMCA. Served on the President's Summit

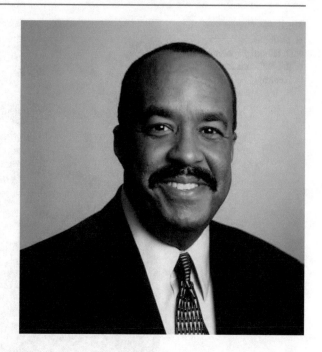

Fig. 6.65 Robert K. Ross, MD. (Photograph courtesy of Dr. Ross)

for America's Future and as chair of the national Boost for Kids Initiative. Named by the Council on Foundations as the Distinguished Grantmaker of the Year for 2008.

31. Gary H. Gibbons, MD (Fig. 6.66) Undergraduate: Princeton University. Medical school: Harvard, magna cum laude. Residency and Cardiology fellowship: Brigham and Women's Hospital and Harvard Medical School. Appointed Director of the National Heart, Lung, and Blood Institute (NHLBI) of the NIH in 2012. Oversees an annual budget of $3 billion and supervises 917 employees. Former faculty member at Stanford University and Harvard Medical School. Prior to his appointment to NHLBI, he established the Cardiovascular Research Institute at Morehouse School of Medicine, which developed into a center of excellence focusing on discoveries related to the cardiovascular health of minorities. He was also Chair of the Physiology Department and Professor of Medicine and Physiology. Elected to the Institute of Medicine (now known as the National Academy of Medicine, one of three academies that make up the US National Academies of Sciences, Engineering, and Medicine) and was a Robert Wood Johnson Foundation Minority Faculty Development Awardee.

32. Paula A. Johnson, MD, MPH (Fig. 6.67) Undergraduate: Harvard and Radcliffe. Medical school and MPH: Harvard Medical School. Residency in Internal Medicine and Cardiology Fellowship: Brigham and Women's Hospital and Harvard Medical School, where she was the first African American chief resident in medicine. Specialty: Cardiology. 14th President of Wellesley College. The first African American to lead that institution. Founder and former Executive Director of the Connors Center for Women's Health and Gender

Fig. 6.66 Gary H. Gibbons, MD. (Photograph courtesy of the National Institutes of Health)

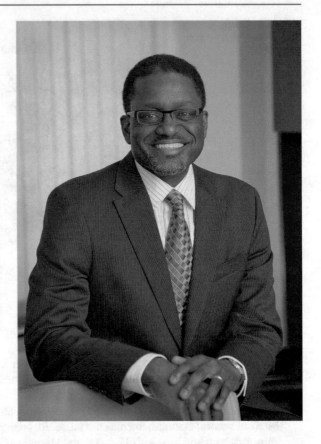

Biology and former Chief, Division of Women's Health, both at Brigham and Women's Hospital, leading research into furthering our knowledge of biological differences between males and females that also resulted in advances in health policy. Former Grayce A. Young Family Professor of Medicine in Women's Health at Harvard Medical School, a professorship named in honor of her mother, and professor of Epidemiology at the Harvard T. H. Chan School of Public Health. The first African American to achieve the rank of professor at Brigham and Women's Hospital. A member of the AAAS and of the National Academy of Medicine. As president of Wellesley, she has advanced women's higher education, championing cross-campus efforts to integrate the ideals of inclusive excellence into the academic program and residential life. With a belief that health and wellness are crucial to fulfilling one's potential, she is reimagining how a college integrates a public health agenda as an essential component of a college education. The College is developing new opportunities by drawing on the synergies found at the intersection of science, the humanities, and social sciences.

Fig. 6.67 Paula
A. Johnson,
MD. (Photograph courtesy
of Dr. Johnson)

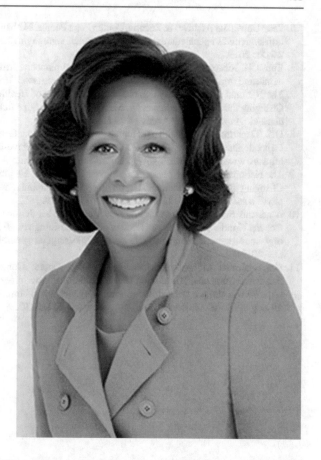

In conclusion, I have made an attempt in this chapter to recognize and give credit to some of the black medical heroes in our country's history. Others are included in other chapters in this book, but I acknowledge that there are still several individuals who are not accounted for. With all respect that is due to them, I give a silent, unwritten tribute to all of them as well as to all who appear on these pages.

References

1. Wynn LT. Robert Fulton Boyd (1855-1912). In: Lovett BL, Wynn LT, editors. African-American members of the Tennessee General Assembly, 1873–1995. http://ww2.tnstate.edu/library/digital/RFBoyd.htm.
2. Dr. Charles Victor Roman. J Natl Med Assoc. 1953;45(4):301–5.
3. Morrison SM, Fee E, Charles V. Roman: physician, writer, educator, historian (1864-1934). Am J Public Health. 2010;100(Suppl 1):S69.
4. Dr. Nathan F. Mossell. Oldest Active Negro Physician, Uncle to Paul Robeson, Was 90. The New York Times. 29 Oct 1946, p. 23.

5. Penn University Archives & Records Center. Penn People. Nathan Francis Mossell. 1856–1946. https://archives.upenn.edu/exhibits/penn-people/biography/nathan-francis-mossell. Accessed 24 Dec 2019.
6. Epps CH, Johson DG. Vaughan Al. Black medical pioneers. African-American 'firsts' in academic and organized medicine. Part three. J Natl Med Assoc. 1993;85(10):777–96.
7. The National Library of Medicine. National Institutes of Health, Health & Human Services, Changing the Face of Medicine. Dr. M. Jocelyn Elders. https://cfmedicine.nlm.nih.gov/physicians/biography_98.html. Accessed 23 Dec 2019.
8. U.S. Department of Health & Human Services. Surgeon General.gov. Previous Surgeons General. David Satcher (1998–2002) http://wayback.archive-it.org/3929/20171201191751/https://www.surgeongeneral.gov/about/previous/biosatcher.html. Accessed 24 Dec 2019.
9. The National Library of Medicine. National Institutes of Health, Health & Human Services, Changing the Face of Medicine. Dr. Regina Marcia Benjamin. https://cfmedicine.nlm.nih.gov/physicians/biography_31.html. Accessed 24 Dec 2019.
10. American Society of Anesthesiologists Congratulates Jerome Adams, M.D., for Surgeon General Nomination. American Society of Anesthesiologists. 29 Jun 2017. https://www.asahq.org/about-asa/newsroom/news-releases/2017/06/surgeon-general-nomination. Accessed 24 Dec 2019.
11. U.S. National Library of Medicine. Opening Doors: Contemporary African American Academic Surgeons. It's attitude, not aptitude, that determines altitude (Claude H. Organ). https://www.nlm.nih.gov/exhibition/aframsurgeons/organ.html. 14 Nov 2006; last reviewed: 19 Aug 2011; last updated 17 Jul 2013. Accessed 24 Dec 2019.

The Importance of Trust in the Physician-Patient Relationship and in Medical Care

7

Introduction

In order for the treatment prescribed by the physician to be effective or even to be utilized by the patient, a tacit bond of *trust* must be established between the two. A contract of trust between physician and patient and articulation of ethical principles of medical treatment were enunciated over 2300 years ago in the Hippocratic Oath and were reiterated centuries later in the Oath of Maimonides. (African American physicians who join the National Medical Association swear to the Oath of Imhotep, the ancient Egyptian physician who was the first person recognized as a doctor in history. The oath was written by Anthony C. Pickett, MD, and published in the *Journal of the National Medical Association* [1]). This issue of trust is of paramount significance as one of the determinants of the efficacy and ethics of healthcare delivery in the United States (US) and throughout the industrialized world. In addition, the American Medical Association Code of Ethics [2] states that building relationships of trust with patients is fundamental to ethical practice in medicine. In this chapter, trust will be examined as a principle regarding how it is perceived by the general public, and then it will be analyzed according to how it is perceived by the African American population.

The Public Perception of Trust

How is trust defined? The *Oxford English Dictionary* defines it as "firm belief based on experience, qualities such as honesty, and veracity, and actions such as justice and strength of a person or thing." It might also be generally described more simply as the expression of confidence in something or someone. Any definition used must be appropriate to the entities being considered. For instance, the issue can refer to the public and its trust of physicians. Another definition that is more relevant to the individual physician-patient relationship is the belief that someone else or another entity will act in your interest in the future [3].

© Springer Nature Switzerland AG 2020
R. A. Williams, *Blacks in Medicine*, https://doi.org/10.1007/978-3-030-41960-8_7

Recent studies and surveys of the level of trust that the American public has for its physicians reveal that the majority of people actually mistrust their physicians [3]. Compared to 29 other industrialized countries surveyed by the International Social Survey Programme (ISSP), the United States ranked near the bottom in terms of level of trust expressed by the public for their physicians. A number of polls in this country over the past several years have shown a steady decline in public trust of physicians. For instance, it was found that the nation's trust of physician leaders declined precipitously over the past half century; in 1966, public confidence in physicians was 73%, but by 2012, the confidence level had fallen to 34% (Harris Poll, 1966–2012). These trends contrast sharply with the public's views of physician integrity, honesty, and ethical standards, which have been consistently high (Gallup Poll, 2013). In addition, although ranking near the bottom of the ISSP list in terms of trust, US physicians rank near the top in patient satisfaction. This paradox is difficult to explain.

Let us review some of the factors that are involved in determining the public's trust of physicians.

The Influence of Level of Income on Trust

Patient income definitely matters when the level of trust is assessed. Those whose income is under $30,000 are the least trusting of physicians and the most dissatisfied with their care. In the ISSP survey, a minority of low-income patients (47%) felt that their physicians could be trusted, compared to 67% in the higher-income group.

Age and Gender as Factors Influencing Trust

The same survey also indicated that level of trust varies by age, with patients over 65 being more trusting than younger ones, and by gender, with men being more trusting than women.

Institutional and System-Wide Determinants of Trust

The American public also does not have a high level of trust for medical institutions such as hospitals and medical schools, and its level of confidence in the healthcare system is extremely low at 23% [4–6].

Special Considerations of Trust

Certain racial and ethnic groups in the United States have had experiences that have formed perceptions of trust that are starkly different from the general public. We will use the black population as an example.

While serving as the 117th president of the National Medical Association (NMA), the largest group of black physicians in the world, I had a unique opportunity to observe and examine the issue of trust as seen through the eyes of African American patients and their physicians. My observations were in addition to the years that I have spent practicing medicine and cardiology. My interest in historical occurrences affecting black people also has served me well in developing a retrospective view of trust for blacks in its entirety that has never been represented before in the medical literature. This presentation is in tribute to the late W. Montague Cobb, MD, PhD, who was a distinguished professor at the esteemed Howard University College of Medicine, a past president of the NMA and the NAACP, a political activist who met several times with US presidents at the Imhotep Conferences at the White House [7] to press the fight for the civil rights of health, and the major historian of blacks in Medicine [8]. He was also a personal mentor for me.

The Tragic Historical Background of Blacks in the United States: A Record of Betrayal of Trust

Black people, called Negroes at that time, arrived in this country in chains in 1619, exactly 400 years ago, 1 year before the Mayflower landed [9] after being transported across the Middle Passage, and were immediately sold into slavery. They had no choice in the selection of the meager amount of medical treatment that they received whenever they fell ill. That treatment was often deficient in its quality and quantity; not much time and money were spent on medical problems of slaves who were needed in the fields and were not allowed to be away from their chores for too long. They soon developed treatments of their own that fall into the category of folk medicine (see Chap. 2). They had to learn to take care of themselves rather than relying on the "white man's medicine" dispensed by their masters and the local physicians that the masters might hire when the illness was serious or severe. The master often purchased insurance on his slaves who were considered a valuable commodity whose disability or demise would result in significant monetary loss. The fact that some of the best-known American insurance companies aided and abetted slavery by selling life insurance policies on slaves raises ethical questions that have not been fully addressed by our society and raises further questions of trust regarding those famous insurance corporations.

There were several miscarriages of justice that affected the trust that blacks have in the medical system and in physicians. Some of the most notorious were the medical escapades of Dr. J. Marion Sims (1813–1883), often called the father of modern gynecology. Between 1846 and 1849, he demonstrated his gynecological experiments on naked black slave women, the best known of whom were named Anarcha, Betsey, and Lucy, in full view of the public and without the use of anesthesia. All were used as human guinea pigs in Sims' monstrous experiments. He traveled around the country with his slave women like the barker at a carnival show (Fig. 7.1). During these expositions, he would demonstrate his technique of repairing vesicovaginal fistulas and how to use the vaginal speculum that he had invented

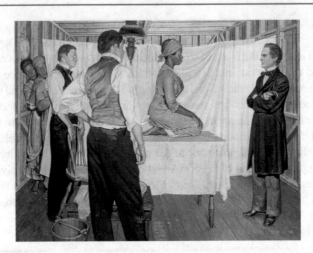

Fig. 7.1 *Illustration of Dr. J. Marion Sims with Anarcha* by Robert Thom. An "experimental" slave woman, she was subjected to 30 surgeries. (This painting by Robert Thom, part of the *Great Moments in Medicine* series, is the only known representation of Lucy, Anarcha, and Betsey, the three enslaved women Sims operated upon. Courtesy of the University of Michigan; from the collection of Michigan Medicine, University of Michigan, Gift of Pfizer, Inc., UMHS.30)

(Fig. 7.2). Many of these women were maimed and some actually died. Despite the fact that many medical authorities condemned the brutality of his experiments, he became a legend in the eyes of American physicians in general, and rather than being rebuked, he was even elected President of the American Medical Association (AMA) in 1876 [10]. He also established the first hospital for women in the United States, Women's Hospital, in New York City, in 1855, where he performed more of his torturous and disfiguring surgeries such as clitoridectomies on women as an alleged cure for hypersexuality. Sims was thrown out of his own hospital in 1874 by his fellow physicians who determined that his work was reckless and lethal. Eventually he became immortalized in stone with the erection of a statue of him in New York City's Central Park (Fig. 7.3), which was removed in April 2018 after numerous objections to his racist history, including a protest from members of the National Medical Association. However, other statues of Sims remain in several US locations, including in his hometown of Lancaster County, South Carolina; at his alma mater, Jefferson Medical College in Philadelphia, PA; at the Alabama State Capital in Montgomery; and at the South Carolina State House in Columbia. Such is his mixed legacy of fame and infamy, in which he has been celebrated as a physician who allegedly brought relief to many women's gynecological ills, including empresses, but also brought pain, suffering, and death to many other women, especially those who could not defend themselves against his horrible experimentation. Based on his racist history, he occupies a seat in the pantheon of evil-doers against black people and is a prime exemplar of mistrust for black people. There is still much work to be done to bring a semblance of justice to the women whom he harmed. It has been suggested that his statue that was removed in New York's Central Park should be replaced with a plaque commemorating his victims of abuse.

Fig. 7.2 Dr. Sims's vaginal speculum. (Public domain, https://commons.wikimedia.org/w/index.php?curid=5328145)

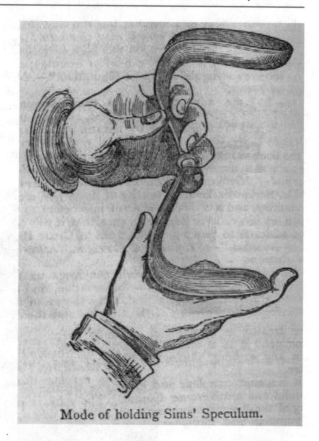

Mode of holding Sims' Speculum.

Fig. 7.3 Statue of J. Marion Sims in New York's Central Park. It was removed in 2018 after numerous protests. (Photograph by Jim Henderson, released to public domain)

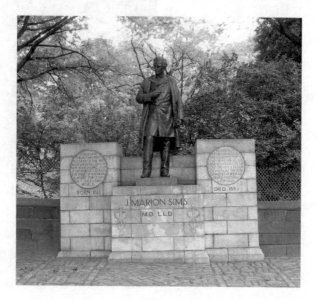

His legacy is one of the principal reasons that blacks have for mistrusting the system of healthcare delivery in this country and why they are very suspicious of participating in clinical research trials.

The story of Henrietta Lacks (1920–1951) (Fig. 7.4) also resonates in the annals of medical history in the United States as an example of why blacks mistrust the medical system. It concerns a black woman who developed cervical cancer in 1951 and was treated at Johns Hopkins Hospital in Baltimore, Maryland. During her treatment, the cancer was biopsied, and the cells from the tumor were cultured to produce what is called an immortal cell line, which means that the cells would

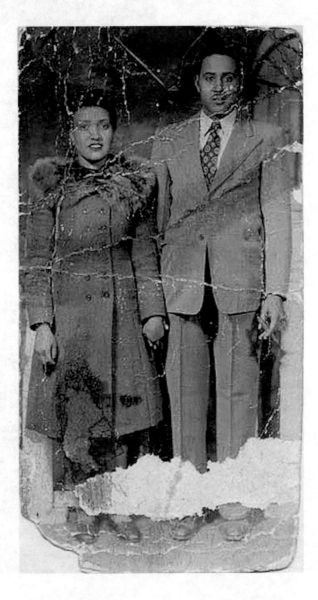

Fig. 7.4 Henrietta Lacks, whose cells were used in human research without permission. (Photograph courtesy of the Lacks family)

reproduce perpetually and could be used indefinitely for experimental research. The researcher and physician who extracted and developed these unique cells from Henrietta Lacks's tissue, Dr. George Otto Gey, named it the HeLa immortal cell line, which was unusual in that they were the first cells that were found to reproduce at a very high rate and to stay alive long enough to allow experimental studies to be completed. HeLa cells are still used in research to this very day; they have been responsible for hundreds of scientific and medical discoveries and have also been employed commercially for financial profit. Unfortunately, Ms. Lacks's permission was not sought for the use of her private biological materials, nor was she or her family credited or financially compensated for this huge contribution to medical science.

Although disclosure protocols and permission for human studies were not standardly used at the time of these developments, many observers are of the opinion that this was an unethical situation and an abuse of human rights and the principles of privacy. Also, according to an article in *The New York Times*, it was not until 1973, when a scientist called to ask Henrietta Lacks's children for blood samples to study the genes they had inherited from her, did the Lacks family learn "that their mother's cells were, in effect, scattered across the planet" [11]. The genetic information of the "immortal" Henrietta Lacks continues to be exploited and made available for public use. As recently as 2013, the genome of a strain of HeLa cells with its DNA sequence was published by researchers without the consent of her surviving family. However, the family has since then gained some control over how her genome will be used, although they will share none of the profit from any resulting research [11].

Thus, the Henrietta Lacks experience has once more for African Americans brought to the fore the abuse of human rights and has provided a rationale for mistrust of medical science. That sentiment was recently accentuated by the award-winning book, *The Immortal Life of Henrietta Lacks*, published in 2009 [12] and the subsequent recent film starring Oprah Winfrey.

The next episode in the "travesty of trust" series is the Tuskegee Syphilis Study. This was the "granddaddy" of all human rights abuses in the United States, and it was conceived, initiated, perpetrated, sustained, and perpetuated by the US government, principally through the US Public Health Service (PHS) and the Centers for Disease Control and Prevention (CDC). It has been called "arguably the most infamous research study in U.S. history" [13].

In 1932, 399 black males with syphilis and a cohort of 201 black men who did not have the disease were recruited into a study centered at Tuskegee University (Fig. 7.5). All of the study subjects were poor black sharecroppers from Macon County, Alabama, and they were told that they would receive free medical care, food, and burial insurance from the US government for participating. The study was allegedly conceived by Taliaferro Clark, who was head of the venereal disease study

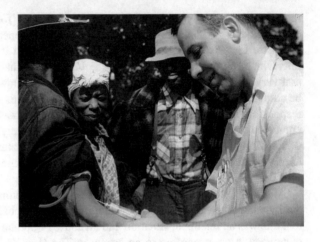

Fig. 7.5 Tuskegee Syphilis Study physician injecting patient. (National Archives Atlanta, GA (U.S. government) - [1], originally from National Archives, Public Domain, https://commons. wikimedia.org/w/index. php?curid=9774274)

group at the PHS national headquarters in 1932 and was carried forward by Dr. Thomas Parran after Clark resigned a year after it began. Dr. Parran was celebrated for his medical expertise and became the sixth US Surgeon General.

The study was designed to follow the victims of the disease untreated to observe its natural history undisturbed and unmodified by any medical treatment. The ultimate goal was to follow the men to their deaths and then to perform autopsies on their bodies to determine what pathological changes were caused by syphilis [14]. This was declared to be for the benefit of humanity. It would continue for 40 years and was stopped only after a whistleblower, Peter Buxton, a former PHS employee, informed *The New York Times* about the unethical experiment in 1972. After the story exploded on the front page of the newspaper, there was widespread condemnation of the study, and attempts were made by government officials as well as those at Tuskegee to explain why it had been allowed to occur in the first place and why the black subjects had been denied available treatment despite the fact that penicillin had been known to be an effective cure for syphilis since 1947. No one wanted to take responsibility for the study, and at the end, there was much assignment of blame and finger-pointing. It was decried as one of the most racist incidents in history and as a prime example of why people could not trust physicians and the government [15]. Years after the study was terminated, Congress decided that some reparations were due the surviving study participants, and $10 million dollars was given to them, which seemed to be a mere pittance for their suffering. A formal apology was also given in person in a public ceremony to some of the survivors by President Bill Clinton on May 17, 1997 (Fig. 7.6).

The Tuskegee Syphilis Study had both positive and negative fallout. On the positive side, federal legislation was passed that mandated the development of informed consent measures that henceforth were used in all scientific investigations involving human subjects. Governmental agencies were opened to establish ethical criteria that had to be applied to determine if a study qualified for performance and which monitored the course of the investigation. Hospitals, clinics, and other medical facilities were required to submit their proposed experiments to Institutional

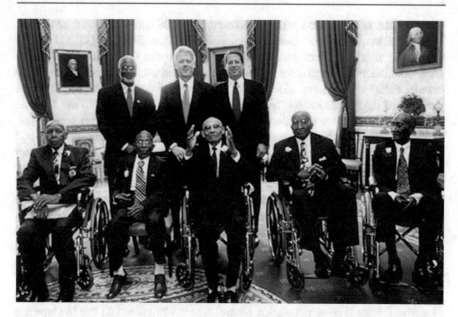

Fig. 7.6 President Bill Clinton apologizing to the participants and survivors of the Tuskegee Syphilis Study on May 16, 1997, on behalf of the US government. (White House Photography Office 1997)

Review Boards (IRBs), which consisted not only of people who had great scientific knowledge but also ordinary citizens and members of the faith community as well as ethicists. On the negative side, the black community took the news of the study as evidence that whites, and the federal government in particular, regarded blacks as subhuman. Mistrust abounded, and visits by blacks to hospitals and physicians' offices decreased. Books were written which described the horrors of the study, such as *Bad Blood* [16] by James Jones. The Tuskegee Syphilis Study was considered by many as onerous in its own way as the Nazi Holocaust with respect to its complete and intentional disregard for human life on a racial or ethnic basis. In later years, when the HIV/AIDS epidemic occurred, which disproportionately affected blacks, there were suspicions in the African American community that this was another plot by the racist white government to eliminate blacks [17]. In addition, the study has had a negative impact on the willingness of blacks to participate in clinical research trials, which are vitally important to document the effectiveness of experimental drugs, devices, and scientific treatment [18].

The Societal Context Surrounding Trust-Losing Events

The end of the nineteenth century and the entire twentieth century have been imbued with an aura of racism that has affected the amount of trust held by African Americans in the federal government, medical institutions, the healthcare system, and physicians. This period began with several legal decisions such as the Supreme Court decision in the trial *Dred Scott v. John F.A. Sandford*, 60 US 393 (1857) (Fig. 7.7), in which Chief Justice Roger Taney and the Court ruled that blacks were not citizens and therefore could not claim freedom, and continued with the case of *Plessy v. Ferguson*, 163 US 537 (1896), a decision in which the Supreme Court ruled that it was lawful for blacks and whites to be required to use separate public facilities such as trains, schools, hospitals, etc., as long as they were equal. These and other edicts instituted, reinforced, and perpetuated discrimination and gave legal status to segregation and inferior medical treatment for blacks. Another aspect of this differential treatment phenomenon was the use of sterilization, which could be court-ordered or performed by obstetricians and gynecologists using their "clinical judgment" to prevent minority group women from having more babies by tying their tubes without their consent. This abhorrent practice against black women was so detested in the South that it received a derisive nickname, the "Mississippi appendectomy." This practice was definitely a form of population control, racial and ethnic cleansing, and eugenics, and it received a great deal of support from social and healthcare conservatives. It is said that Adolf Hitler so admired the practice of sexual sterilization that was rampant in California in the 1930s that he used it as an incentive for the type of population control that the Nazis would use in Germany (California led all states with 20,000 such procedures!) [19, 20].

Because of this practice and other examples of racial and ethnic disregard, an aura of mistrust was created that has continued to the present time. It set the stage for the civil rights struggles of the 1930s and 1940s that culminated in the activities, protests, marches, and civil disobedience involving Rev. Dr. Martin Luther King, Jr. and his followers and associates. An underlying political counterculture developed that involved the highest levels of the US government attempting to hold African Americans back from advancing their civil rights agenda. The Federal Bureau of Investigation (FBI) was a participant in much of this counteractivity [18]. In addition, during the Nixon administration, the so-called War on Drugs was declared in 1971, ostensibly to eliminate the narcotics abuses that have been running rampant in this country. All of the forces of the federal government were trained on this mission, which continued through the Reagan administration, when it reached its peak in incarcerations in 1981. In actual fact, this was a "War on Blacks," as evidenced by the fact that over 80% of those prosecuted and given long prison terms for possession of crack cocaine were members of that particular racial group.

Dr. King was one of the individuals most heavily persecuted during this period of attempted civil rights oppression, along with several other black activists. Much of this selective attention given to black activists came at the hands of the FBI, which was found in 1971 to have a secret agency that was vicious in its pursuit of black activists [21]. Called COINTELPRO (Counterintelligence Program), it was supposed to have been formed to fight communism in the United States, but in fact, its actual main mission was to attempt to destroy African American dissent and black people's push for justice through the use of strong-arm tactics, intimidation, and murder, such as the illegal raid on Black Panther Party headquarters in Chicago in 1969 where two leaders of the "BPP," as FBI Director J. Edgar Hoover called it,

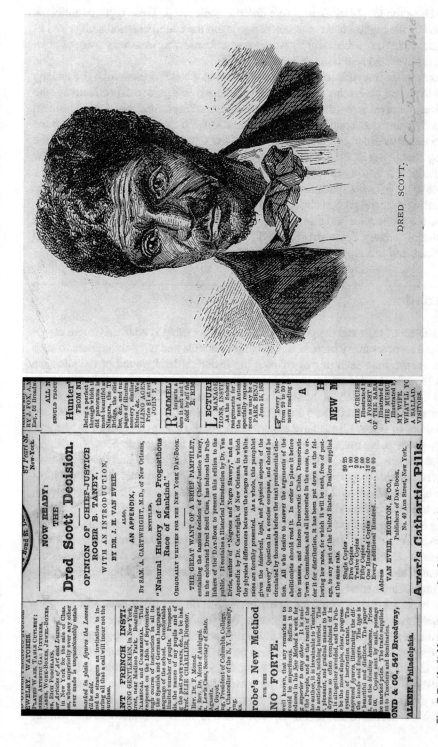

Fig. 7.7 (*Left*) Newspaper notice for a pamphlet on the US Supreme Court's Dred Scott decision. Illustration in Harper's Weekly, v. 3, no, 134, July 23, 1859, page 479. (Courtesy Library of Congress, Washington D. C., ng. No. LC-USZ62-132561). (*Right*) Dred Scott. Print published in Century Magazine, June 1887. (Courtesy Library of Congress, Washington, D.C. Control Number 2014645331)

Fred Hampton and Mark Clark, were killed in their sleep. These types of antiblack actions by the highest law enforcement agency in the country caused a huge loss of confidence in the government by African Americans, who were very wary of placing their lives and health in the hands of whites.

Some relief from this terrible pressure occurred when President John F. Kennedy came to power; his brother Robert (Bobby) Kennedy was particularly effective as the Attorney General in putting down segregation and discrimination. After President Kennedy was assassinated in 1963, President Lyndon Baines Johnson took up the battle and succeeded in gaining passage of the Civil Rights Act in 1964 and the Voting Rights Act in 1965, with Medicare and Medicaid also being signed into law by President Johnson, who said pointedly, "And we shall overcome" at the end of a speech to the joint houses of Congress and to the nation, 1 week after violence broke out during peaceful protests by African Americans in Selma, Alabama.

Such actions gave some impetus to those seeking civil liberties and justice in healthcare delivery, but mistrust of medical authorities still loomed like a dark cloud overhead, and this atmosphere of mistrust continues to this day.

Conclusion

The subject of trust and the physician-patient relationship is obviously more extensive and involves many more issues than how patients and physicians relate to each other. As we have seen in this chapter, the historical background of the situation must be understood if we are to be able to improve upon what is currently a bad situation that can definitely be harmful to the welfare of the patients whom we serve. There is no doubt that there is an overlap between societal and historical events and the loss of trust that blacks have experienced. As medical practitioners and healthcare providers, we must develop more opportunities for dialogue between patients and physicians, medical institutions, and government agencies and between stakeholders and gatekeepers to attempt to rebuild and regain the trust that people must have in those who would treat them. Providers and institutions must do a better job in creating trust with individual patients than has been done before. This will require going beyond mere facts and beyond evidence base to seek the real truth [20]. Such a step is important to dispel the current mistrust in science that threatens the patient-physician relationship [22]. This is especially important for the African American, Hispanic, and other minority populations who have endured healthcare disparities that impact their survival.

A good beginning would be to link trust to truth and transparency in the government's intentions in bringing about truly effective and universal healthcare for the American people. We must speak truth to power as we explore deeper into the evolving genomic science, ostensibly to utilize biomedical information in a translational and humane fashion and to bring the wonderful capabilities and medical discoveries that are developed for the public benefit. We must be careful not to allow the people's trust to be betrayed again as has been done so frequently in the past. With specific regard to blacks, there needs to be an assurance that the mantras of "never again" and "black lives matter" are believable. Wisdom drawn from our past experiences dictates that a nongovernmental watchdog or monitoring group should be established that reports progress and use of data derived from experimental genomic programs—such as the National Institutes of Health *All of Us* research program (https://allofus.nih.gov/about/scientific-opportunities)—back to the public on a regular basis. That may help to rebuild, regain, and maintain the public's trust in medicine and healthcare.

References

1. Pickett AC. The oath of Imhotep: in recognition of African contributions to Western medicine. J Natl Med Assoc. 1992;84(7):636–7.
2. American Medical Association. AMA code of medical ethics. https://www.ama-assn.org/topics/ama-code-medical-ethics.
3. Hardin R. Conceptions and explanations of trust. In: Cook K, editor. Trust in society, vol. 2. New York: Russell Sage Foundation; 2001. p. 3–40.
4. Blendon RJ, Benson JM, Hero JO. Public trust in physicians—U. S. medicine in international perspective. N Engl J Med. 2014;371(17):1570–2.
5. Buhr T, Blendon RJ. Trust in government and health care institutions. In: Blendon RJ, Brodie M, Benson JM, Altman DE, editors. American public opinion and health care. Washington, DC: CQ Press; 2011. p. 15–38.
6. Hetherington MJ. Why trust matters: declining political trust and the demise of American liberalism. Princeton: Princeton University Press; 2005.
7. Cobb WM. The White House conference "to fulfill these rights". The ninth Imhotep conference. J Natl Med Assoc. 1966;58(4):292–passim.
8. Sampson CC. William Montague Cobb MD, PhD 1904-1990. J Natl Med Assoc. 1991;83(1):13–4.
9. Bennett L Jr. Before the Mayflower: a history of black America: the classic account of the struggles and triumphs of black Americans. New York: Penguin Books; 1961.
10. Spettel S, White MD. The portrayal of J. Marion Sims' controversial surgical legacy. J Urol. 2011;185(6):2424–7.
11. Zimmer C. A family consents to a medical gift, 62 years later. The New York Times, 8 Aug 2013, Section A, Page 1. https://www.nytimes.com/2013/08/08/science/after-decades-of-research-henrietta-lacks-family-is-asked-for-consent.htmln. 8 Aug 2013.
12. Skloot R. The immortal life of Henrietta Lacks. New York: Crown; 2009.
13. Katz RV, Kegeles SS, Kressin NR, Green BL, Wang MQ, James SA, et al. The Tuskegee legacy project: willingness of minorities to participate in biomedical research. J Health Care Poor Underserved. 2006;17(4):698–715.
14. Brandt AM. Racism and research: the case of the Tuskegee Syphilis Study. Hastings Cent Rep. 1978;8(6):21–9.
15. Jones J, Tuskegee Institute. Bad blood: the Tuskegee syphilis experiment. New York/London: Free Press/Collier Macmillan Publishers; 1981.
16. Thomas SB, Quinn SC. The Tuskegee Syphilis Study, 1932 to 1972: implications for HIV education and AIDS risk education programs in the black community. Am J Public Health. 1991;81(11):1498–505.
17. Katz RV, Green BL, Kressin NR, Kegeles SS, Wang MQ, James SA, et al. The legacy of the Tuskegee Syphilis Study: assessing its impact on willingness to participate in biomedical studies. J Health Care Poor Underserved. 2008;19(4):1168–80.
18. Molina N. Fit to be citizens? Public health and race in Los Angeles, 1879-1939. Berkeley/Los Angeles: University of California Press; 2006.

19. Stern AM. Eugenic nation. Faults & frontiers of better breeding in modern America. Oakland: University of California Press; 2016.
20. Chang S, Lee TH. Beyond evidence-based medicine. N Engl J Med. 2018;379(21):1983–5.
21. Kayyali D. The history of surveillance and the black community. Electronic Frontier Foundation. 13 Feb 2014. https://www.eff.org/deeplinks/2014/02/history-surveillance-and-black-community. Accessed 5 Nov 2019.
22. Baron RJ, Berinsky AJ. Mistrust in science—a threat to the patient-physician relationship. N Engl J Med. 2019;381(2):182–5.

Current Health Status of Blacks in the United States: The Case for Future Improvement of Healthcare Delivery

8

I'm sick and tired of being sick and tired.

—Fannie Lou Hamer
Black civil rights, voting rights, and human rights activist from
Mississippi (1917–1977)

Introduction

The health of black people in the United States is an ever-evolving situation. Information that was pertinent 10 years ago has changed significantly, and it is safe to say that there is always good news and bad news no matter what window we use to view African American health. As time has passed, unfavorable socioeconomic conditions have deeply impacted the third largest racial/ethnic group in the country to the extent that healthcare disparities have continued to lead to higher mortality and greater morbidity for blacks from most major illnesses and diseases compared to other subpopulations. The evidence of these devastating effects is collected by several reliable sources and is produced on a periodic basis that allows us to access the metrics used to follow the trends and perhaps to make some decisions about how to correct the problems that are observed. In this chapter, a compendium of information on health of the African American population entitled *Vital Signs*, produced by the Centers for Disease Control and Prevention (CDC), is used as a basis for indicating those trends and identifying those problems. The chapter that follows this one will address possible solutions to the problems.

© Springer Nature Switzerland AG 2020
R. A. Williams, *Blacks in Medicine*, https://doi.org/10.1007/978-3-030-41960-8_8

Comparative Vital Statistics for Blacks and Whites

We begin by considering the timespan between 1999 and 2015 and looking at the causes of death or mortality figures for blacks compared to whites for the leading diseases in the United States for all ages including children and according to adult age categories (18–34, 35–49, 50–64, ≥65) [1] (Fig. 8.1).

Using 1999 as the comparator year, it is seen that in that year the age-adjusted all-cause death rates were 1135.7 for blacks and 854.6 for whites per 100,000 each. By 2015, those rates had fallen for each group, to 851.9 per 100,000 for blacks and 735.0 per 100,000 for whites. This means that not only have death rates for the major diseases declined for both groups but also the decline for blacks was almost twice as great as for whites, 25% versus 14%, respectively. This also indicates that health disparities, i.e., differences in disease status between these two racial groups, have decreased significantly although a substantial mortality gap favoring whites over blacks remains. Interestingly, however, there was actually a "crossover" beginning in 2010 when blacks in the >65 age category had lower death rates than whites (see Fig. 8.1).

Regarding life expectancy at birth, a comparison between blacks and whites for the years 2000 and 2014 showed that blacks improved from an average of 71.8–75.6 years, an increase of 3.8 years across the 15-year span. This was significantly better than for whites, who improved from an average of 77.3–79.0 years, an increase of 1.7 years. A more recent version of this National Center for Health

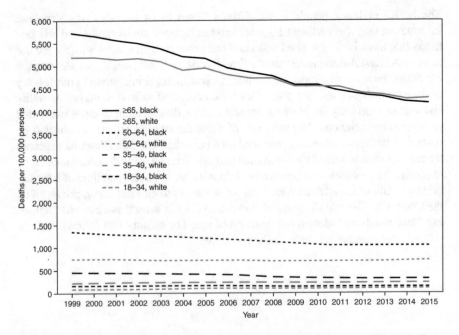

Fig. 8.1 Comparison of death rates between blacks and whites by age group, 1999–2015. (From Cunningham et al. [1])

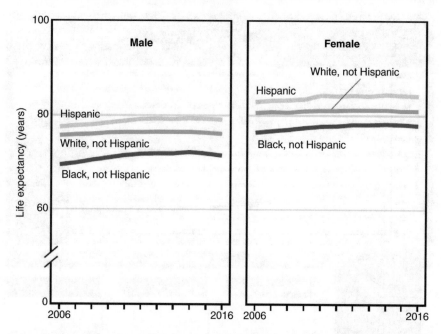

Fig. 8.2 Life expectancy at birth, by sex, race, and Hispanic origin: United States, 2006–2016. (For data table see: https://www.cdc.gov/nchs/hus/contents2017.htm#Figure_001. Note that persons of Hispanic origin can be of any race. Notes: Life expectancy data by Hispanic origin were available starting in 2006 and were corrected to address racial and ethnic misclassification. Life expectancy estimates for 2016 are based on preliminary Medicare data. Source: NCHS. *Health, United States, 2017*, Figure 1. Data from the National Vital Statistics System (NVSS), Mortality)

Statistics report [2] shows a comparison between non-Hispanic blacks and non-Hispanic whites between the years 2006 and 2016, which also demonstrates the same trends, with blacks improving more than whites over that time period (Fig. 8.2).

If we look strictly at differences in health status between blacks and whites during the stated time period, blacks reported that they had fair or poor health compared to whites across all ages. Although there was a disease-specific decline in selected causes of death for blacks during 1999–2015, they still had higher prevalence rates than whites for most serious diseases including heart disease, asthma, diabetes, stroke, and high blood pressure (Fig. 8.3). Cancer was the only major disease group in which prevalence was greater in whites than in blacks.

Death rate differences between blacks and whites are of particular interest. An example is 2015, when *blacks had 40% higher all-cause death rates than whites for all ages under 65*. This is a tremendous disparity. In addition, *deaths have begun to occur at younger ages in blacks, particularly for cancer, heart disease, cerebrovascular disease, diabetes, and homicide* (Fig. 8.4). This is consistent with the fact that *chronic diseases such as type II diabetes which traditionally has been seen primarily in older individuals are occurring years earlier, and patients may have suffered serious organ damage before the disease is detected.* Much of this late awareness may be due to socioeconomic factors; blacks were less likely to see a doctor or to

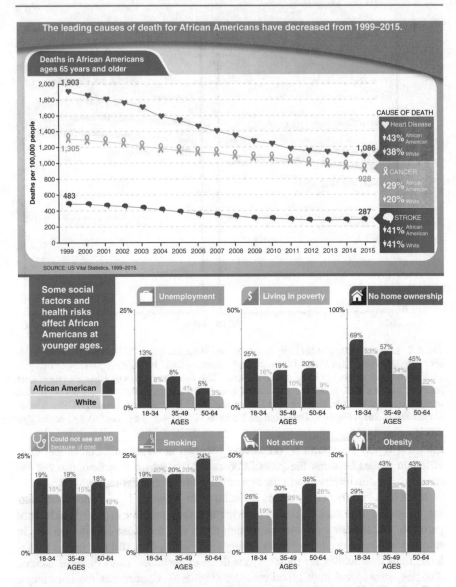

Fig. 8.3 Decrease in death rates for blacks, 1999–2015, and social factors and health risks affecting African Americans. (Courtesy Centers for Disease Control and Prevention Vital Signs. African American Health. https://www.cdc.gov/vitalsigns/aahealth/infographic.html#graphic. Sources: Behavioral Risk Factor Surveillance System, 2015: American Community Survey of the US Census Bureau, 2014)

have a personal physician than whites because of cost [1], and Fig. 8.4 indicates several other factors that may be partly responsible for the increased health risks faced by blacks.

Epidemiology is a powerful and previously underutilized tool for assessing health status, as is geographic location. Recent studies [3–5] have shown that a shift

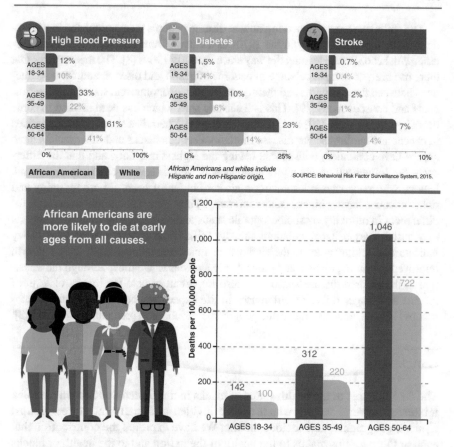

Fig. 8.4 Blacks die at younger ages than whites from all causes. (Courtesy Centers for Disease Control and Prevention Vital Signs. African American Health. https://www.cdc.gov/vitalsigns/aahealth/infographic.html#graphic. Source: US Vital Statistics, 2015)

in leading causes of death is occurring; cancer is replacing heart disease as the mortality leader in the United States and is expected to be the number one cause of *death* by 2020 [6]. Much of this change is attributable to socioeconomic factors as well as racial, ethnic, income, educational, and lifestyle elements. Christopher Murray and his associates described an epidemiological construct called Eight Americas [7] which was an analysis of eight separate subpopulation groups according to distinct geographic, socioeconomic, political, and demographic factors; they discovered that the greatest determinant of disparities in mortality between these eight groups was in their differences in risk factors for chronic diseases such as obesity, smoking, alcohol use, diabetes, and high blood pressure. Race was also an important determinant, but no one factor was dominant. These researchers found that gaps in life expectancy persist despite improvements in healthcare disparities. They feel that the most important and promising interventions involve better treatment and prevention of conditions such as cancer, heart disease, liver cirrhosis, lung disease, and diabetes.

The shifts that we are observing now in disease patterns were articulated in the epidemiologic transition theory in the 1970s as a change from infectious to chronic disease, with heart disease leading the way since the early 1900s [8]. The theory states that there has been "a complex change in patterns of health and disease, and…the interactions between these patterns and their demographic, economic and sociologic determinants and consequences" [9]. This is a seismic shift which has been studied in some detail by Omran et al. [10] and Hastings et al. [11]. Their data showed that disparities in cancer and cardiovascular disease mortality between blacks and other racial/ethnic groups have continued, with blacks having the highest mortality, and that the differences are influenced by county of residence as well as several other socioeconomic factors, with poorer counties having a greater burden of heart disease mortality and richer counties having higher cancer mortality. They state that "failure to account for differences in mortality by socioeconomic status and race/ethnicity in national reports may further marginalize populations already at risk for certain diseases or death." They indicate that taking note of the findings in this observational study could inform improved research, policies, and clinical care agendas as we move through the transition in the chronic disease space. It is also important to note the impact of level of income as a major driver of differences in life expectancy between population subgroups [11] and, as stated, racial and geographic variations in premature mortality [12].

Conclusion

The determinants of the health status of blacks in the United States are a complex mixture of several factors which can be divided artificially into three groups: clinical, geographic, and socioeconomic. We have explored the contribution that each of these groups makes to the health of the nation and to the health of blacks in particular. In view of the fact that the United States spent a staggering $3.5 trillion dollars in 2017 on healthcare costs for 325 million citizens, which amounts to $10,000 per person and 18% of the gross domestic product [13], one would assume that such a large amount of money would result in greater access to care, increased quality of care, and more healthcare equity. However, the evidence indicates otherwise: cardiovascular deaths have recently increased [14]; the country is being roiled by the opioid crisis [15]; obesity, which is linked to several comorbidities such as diabetes and cancer, is highly prevalent and is found more frequently in blacks and Hispanics [16]; and, most importantly, there has been a recent decline in overall life expectancy [17]. In addition, despite the fact that more people are covered by health insurance than at any other time in our history because of the Affordable Care Act, which has been in effect since 2010, according to the Commonwealth Fund, 15.5% of the American working-age population is still uninsured [18]. Paradoxically, despite these problems and others, the health status of blacks has shown some improvement compared to whites, but as has been stated, a substantial distance in health status remains between the two population groups. We must use the considerable resources that this country has to offer to close that gap. The data that has been generated in the various studies, investigations, analyses, and reports referenced above can inform public policy which hopefully will adjust appropriately to correct these problems. Literally hundreds of thousands of lives which depend on access, quality, and equity in healthcare delivery are at stake.

References

1. Cunningham TJ, Croft JB, Liu Y, Lu H, Eke PI, Giles WH. Vital signs: racial disparities in age-specific mortality among blacks or African Americans—United States, 1999-2015. MMWR Morb Mortal Wkly Rep. 2017;66(17):444–56. Erratum: MMWR Morb Mortal Wkly Rep. 2017;66(18):490.
2. National Center for Health Statistics. Health, United States. 2017: with special feature on mortality. Hyattsville; 2018.
3. Colby SL, Ortman JM. Projections of the size and composition of the U. S. population: 2014 to 2060. Washington, DC: U.S. Department of Commerce, Economics and Statistics and Administration, Bureau of the Census; 2014.
4. Heron M, Anderson RN. Changes in the leading cause of death: recent patterns in heart disease and cancer mortality. NCHS Data Brief. 2016;254:1–8.
5. Twombly R. Cancer surpasses heart disease as leading cause of death in all but the very elderly. J Natl Cancer Inst. 2005;97(5):330–1.
6. Krieger N, Rehkopf DH, Chen JT, Waterman PD, Marcelli E, Kennedy M. The fall and rise of US inequities in premature mortality: 1960-2002. PLoS Med. 2008;5(2):e46.
7. Weir HK, Anderson RN, Coleman King SM, Soman A, Thompson TD, Hong Y, et al. Heart disease and cancer deaths—trends and projections in the United States, 1969-2020. Prev Chron Dis. 2016;13:E157.
8. Murray CJ, Kulkarni SC, Michaud C, Tomijima N, Buzacchelli MT, Iandioro TJ, Ezzati M. Eight Americas: investigating mortality disparities across races, counties, and race-counties in the United States. PLoS Med. 2006;3(9):e260.
9. National Center for Health Statistics. Leading causes of death, 1900–1998. Atlanta: Centers for Disease Control and Prevention; 2008.
10. Omran AR. The epidemiologic transition. A theory of the epidemiology of population change. Milbank Mem Fund Q. 1971;49(4):509–38.
11. Hastings KG, Boothroyd DB, Kapphan K, Hu J, Rehkopf DH, Cullen MR, Palaniappan L. Socioeconomic differences in the epidemiologic transition from heart disease to cancer as the leading cause of death in the United States, 2003 to 2015: an observational study. Ann Intern Med. 2018;169(12):836–44.
12. Chetty R, Stepner M, Abraham S, Lin S, Scuderi B, Turner N, et al. The association between income and life expectancy in the United States, 2001-2014. JAMA. 2016;315(16):1750–66.
13. Cullen MR, Cummins C, Fuchs VR. Geographic and racial variation in premature mortality in the U.S.: analyzing the disparities. PLoS One. 2012;7:e32930.
14. Centers for Medicare and Medicaid Services. National Health Expenditure Fact Sheet. https://www.cms.gov/Research-Statistics-Data-and-Systems-Trends-and-Reports/NationalHealthExpendData/NHE-Fact-Sheet.html. Accessed 20 Dec 2019.
15. Benjamin EJ, Muntner P, Alonso A, Bittencourt MS, Callaway CW, Carson AP, et al. American Heart Association Council on Epidemiology and Prevention Statistics Committee and Stroke Statistics Subcommittee. Heart disease and stroke statistics −2019 update: a report from the American Heart Association. Circulation. 2019;139(10):e56–e528.
16. Gomes T, Tadrous M, Mamdani MM, Paterson JM, Juurlink DN. The burden of opioid-related mortality in the United States. JAMA Netw Open. 2018;1(2):e180217.

17. Hales CM, Fryar CD, Carroll MD, Freedman DS, Aoki Y, Ogden CL. Trends in obesity and severe obesity prevalence in US youth and adults by sex and age, 2007-2008 to 2015-2016. JAMA. 2018;319(16):1723–5.
18. Collins SR, Gunja MZ, Doty MM, Buhupal HK. First look at health insurance coverage in 2018 finds ACA gains beginning to reverse. The Commonwealth Fund. To the Point. 1 May 2018. https://www.commonwealthfund.org/blog/2018/first-look-health-insurance-coverage-2018-finds-aca-gains-beginning-reverse.

The Socioeconomic Determinants of Health and Their Impact on African American Healthcare Delivery

Introduction

This chapter deals with what many consider the most important cause of the health problems suffered by blacks and other minorities in the United States. A precise definition of the *socioeconomic determinants of health* is difficult to describe in a brief statement, but it may be generally thought of as those factors that derive from unhealthy conditions that exist where people live, work, and play. Some would describe it as the sum total of negative health-related factors that impinge upon a person in his or her environment, which includes poor housing, inferior wages, contaminated drinking water (think of Flint, Michigan), substandard hospitals, lack of sufficient recreational and educational facilities, etc. Whatever definition that is used is bound to be wanting, because there are myriad causes of this phenomenon; it is truly indescribable, and as it is said, it is hard to get one's arms around it. The World Health Organization (WHO) attempted a definition which is "the conditions into which people are born, grow, live, work, and age"; according to Byyny, this involves complex interactions between economic, lifestyle, environmental, biological, and social factors that affect well-being and health [1]. In addition, since place of residence has emerged as a major determinant of health status as well as longevity, it may be said that the zip code may be more important than the genetic code [2], which has implications as to where we should seek solutions to help to eliminate healthcare disparities: not in our genes but in our surroundings.

Historical Background of the Social Determinants of Health (SDH)

Perhaps the most historically significant example of the impact of environmental factors on health occurred in 1854 in London when a cholera epidemic was raging and was killing thousands of people. This was prior to the discovery of infectious pathogens and the development of the germ theory of disease etiology.

© Springer Nature Switzerland AG 2020
R. A. Williams, *Blacks in Medicine*, https://doi.org/10.1007/978-3-030-41960-8_9

No one knew what was causing this deadly scourge or how to deal with it. Dr. John Snow, a physician in London who at the time attempted to treat patients with the disease, conceived the genius idea of tracking its victims as to where they went to obtain water, and by constructing what were called "ghost maps," he determined that many were getting their water from a common source, the Broad Street pump. He convinced city officials to remove the pump handle, rendering the pump useless, and a dramatic reduction in cholera cases ensued. This might be considered the beginning of epidemiology and the mapping of disease occurrence [3].

Description, Documentation, and Impact of SDH

Social determinants of health are becoming recognized more and more as a discrete entity on the healthcare scene (Fig. 9.1) [4] and are now considered to have more gravitas than factors such as access to care in their impact on overall population health (Fig. 9.2) and risk of premature death [5]. One example of the impact that various SDH factors may have on black health is seen in an analysis of racial segregation; it is estimated that *segregation is responsible for 176,000 deaths per year in the United States* [6]. Racial and ethnic residential segregation (RERS) has been identified as a root cause of this phenomenon and has been determined to be a fundamental public health issue which demands resolution. RERS is linked to poverty and can lead to poor health [7].

Fig. 9.1 Contribution of social, economic, and environmental factors to health outcomes. County Health Rankings Model © 2014 UWPHI [4]. (Courtesy and with permission of the University of Wisconsin Population Health Institute. County Health Rankings & Roadmaps 2019. Kaiser Family Foundation. https://www.countyhealthrankings.org. Source: Schroeder [5])

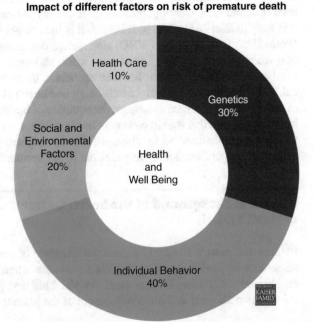

Impact of different factors on risk of premature death

Health Care 10%

Genetics 30%

Social and Environmental Factors 20%

Health and Well Being

Individual Behavior 40%

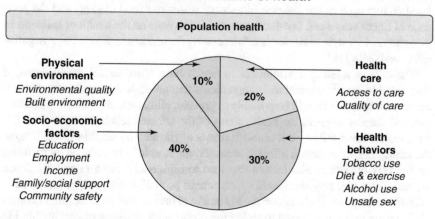

Fig. 9.2 How different factors affect the risk of premature death [5]. (Source: Author's analysis and adaption from the University of Wisconsin Population Health Institute's *County Health Rankings* model ©2010, https://www.countyhealthrankings.org/about-project/background)

The global burden of disease (GBD) study (http://www.healthdata.org/gbd) was initiated in 1990 by Murray and colleagues as an international survey and analysis of illness which uses geographical, sociological, economic, and epidemiological metrics to measure outcomes. It contains a focused investigation on diseases, mortality, morbidity, and longevity in the United States, which identifies major health disparities on a state by state basis. The most recent study, GBD 2016, carried out by Mokdad et al. [8], indicated that 60% of the variation in life expectancy across counties in the United States is related to socioeconomic factors and those related to race and ethnicity.

Linkage of specific disease entities to SDH is in its early stages of development. One area that is being explored extensively is cardiovascular disease (CVD), especially with regard to its association with what is called neighborhood socioeconomic status (nSES), which is a major social determinant of health [9]. A number of investigations have firmly established the association of nSES with general or overall cardiovascular health [10, 11], and there are several studies that have shown its association with specific types of CVD, including stroke [12], heart failure [13], and myocardial infarction [14].

So-called food deserts (FD) and food swamps, which are areas characterized by low access to high-quality healthful foods, such as fresh fruits and vegetables, as well as being low-income areas, have been found to have a higher burden of risk factors for cardiovascular disease. This is where 23.5 million people reside in the United States, including large numbers of blacks and other minorities [15]. If we examine the relationship between living in a food desert and heart failure, which results in over one million hospitalizations a year at a cost to the nation of $15 billion dollars per year [16], we find that there is documentation of such an association, with a very high risk of hospitalization and increased mortality being found in FD areas [17]. This vividly demonstrates the impact that environmental and neighborhood factors such as the absence of grocery stores and food markets and the presence of liquor stores and fast-food restaurants can have on the health of residents in these areas. Lifestyle behavior is influenced by these factors, which has a negative effect on health [18].

These facts relating environment to health have translational implications; if poor neighborhoods contain toxic ingredients that are linked to morbidity, disability, and mortality, it should be possible to prevent, eliminate, or diminish those factors and thereby improve the health status of the affected residents. Specifically, if we consider heart failure as a problem that is aggravated by neighborhood factors, the rehospitalization rate in affected areas should be able to be reduced by focusing on the very environmental factors that lead to high readmission rates [19]. Since we now know that neighborhoods which consist primarily of poor racial and ethnic minorities are more likely to contain FD and to experience adverse health outcomes [20], we are better positioned to tackle the problem by reducing or eliminating FD as a causative factor. This will require collaboration between public health agencies and private entities such as supermarket owners and food manufacturers to control this problem. Health educators and nutritionists also have a role to play in changing and improving this unhealthful scenario. In as much as GBD 2016 referenced above indicates that among mortality risk factors, dietary factors rank number one, it behooves us as a nation to take the steps necessary to resolve this dire situation.

Possible Solutions to the Negative Impact of the Social Determinants of Health

It may be an oversimplification to say that the remedy for adverse SDH effects on the population of the United States lies in more collaboration between federal agencies that oversee housing, education, transportation, and the environment. However, that is essentially what is implied in GBD 2016: our fragmented government services, which consist of silos that operate independent of each other, need to come together to seek common ground in addressing these issues [21]. The National Academy of Medicine also advocates interdisciplinary and cross-sectional collaborations which are expected to lead to more efficient and less costly operations [22]. Our nation also has a disconnect between spending on direct healthcare services and on social services which places us in an inferior position regarding metrics such as life expectancy, in which the United States ranks 43rd among industrialized countries despite the fact that we have the highest per capita health spending rates in the world [23]. This embarrassing phenomenon is known as the *American paradox* [24].

Disease prevention is another dimension where solutions to the adversities of SDH can be sought. A National Prevention Strategy, based on principles drawn from Healthy People 2020, was drafted by Dr. Howard Koh when he was Assistant Secretary for Health for the US Department of Health and Human Services, but unfortunately it did not become an important part of healthcare reform. The Prevention and Public Health Fund also has not lived up to its promise [25]. We must do more as a nation to pay serious attention to preventing disease, which has the potential of saving many lives and so much money.

In order to save lives and money, it will be necessary for the US government to expend more funds on social services. Despite the fact that the United States spends more on healthcare than any other country on the planet, in excess of $3 trillion dollars annually, we have worse outcomes from medical interventions and treatment than almost all of the other industrialized nations. The United States is a member of the Organisation for Economic Co-operation and Development (OECD). Expenditures for healthcare in the United States are 2.5 times more than the average spending by other members of this group, but despite this robust spending, which amounts to almost 18% of our gross domestic product, America occupies the lowest ranks of OECD nations in several measures of health and in life expectancy [26].

To remedy this paradoxical situation, we need to switch our priorities from addressing individual-level health problems to a broader, more comprehensive approach that deals with population health and socioeconomic determinants. Much of the $176.1 billion dollars spent annually in this country on biomedical research should be redirected from biomedical to population pursuits [27]. In this manner, by changing our policies and priorities, we can reduce healthcare disparities more at the neighborhood level and bring more benefits to communities of color [28, 29]. It is time to realign our sights and to aim for greater gains for our population. This will require development of an integrative model of science in which biological research is conducted alongside of investigations into socioeconomic and political determinants of health in an interdisciplinary fashion. In order to accomplish this, the entire structure of the National Institutes of Health will need to be reconfigured from its current focus on individual disease entities into an institution that focuses on collaborative efforts to accomplish broader healthcare objectives so desperately needed by our country [30].

As indicated above and as has been documented, definite illness can arise from the disadvantaged social context [31]. Residing in a disadvantaged neighborhood is associated with higher rates of diseases such as diabetes, cancer, cardiovascular disease, and others, as well as decreased longevity [32, 33]. Therefore, it is very important to have an instrument that can measure the extent of disadvantage in neighborhoods in order for preventive interventions to be made. A research team led by Dr. Amy J.H. Kind at the University of Wisconsin School of Medicine and Public Health has developed a Neighborhood Atlas created from data using their neighborhood-disadvantage metric as a new tool for incorporating data into policy, research, and health interventions [34]. They use the Area Deprivation Index (ADI) that was developed years ago by the Health Resources and Services Administration (HRSA) as well as data derived from the American Community Survey (ACS) to construct a tool that can be used to measure disadvantage as applied to discrete neighborhoods. This ACS-derived ADI is now available for public use for free, and data can be downloaded from the University of Wisconsin website at https://www.neighborhoodatlas.medicine.wisc.edu/. This is the type of research that is needed to move the nation forward in tackling the difficult problems that are caused by the socioeconomics of health.

Conclusion

The subject of the social determinants of health is a new item in the conversation about healthcare disparities, health inequities, and population health, but I believe that it will soon take its rightful place at the top of the list as the most important ingredient in that discussion. As I have indicated, a sweeping, fundamental change in health policy must occur that will allow programs to be developed that will impact on SDH and make it possible to focus on disease prevention and wellness at the neighborhood level, where it is needed the most. This change in health policy must be accompanied by adequate and appropriate funding, which should come from government as well as private sources. Funding support should be provided for community-based research and development of tools such as the neighborhood-disadvantage metric devised by the University of Wisconsin and the application of these tools for the public benefit. That will truly be the proper practice and implementation of public health.

References

1. Byyny RL. Social determinants of health: reforming education and public health to improve health in the United States. The Pharos. Autumn 2017; p. 2–7. http://alphaomegaalpha.org/pharos/2017/Autumn/2017-4-Byyny.pdf.
2. Dwyer-Lindgren L, Bertozzi-Villa A, Stubbs RW, Morozoff C, Mackenbach JP, van Lenthe FJ, et al. Inequalities in life expectancy among US counties, 1980 to 2014: temporal trends and key drivers. JAMA Intern Med. 2017;177(7):1003–11.
3. Johnson S. The ghost map: the story of London's most terrifying epidemic—and how it changed science, cities, and the modern world. New York: Riverhead; 2006.
4. University of Wisconsin Population Health Institute and the Robert Wood Johnson Foundation. County Health Rankings Model. https://www.countyhealthrankings.org/explore-health-rankings/measures-data-sources/county-health-rankings-model. Accessed 17 Oct 2019.
5. Schroeder SA. Shattuck Lecture. We can do better—improving the health of the American people. NEJM. 2007;357(12):1221–8.
6. Galea S, Tracy M, Hoggatt KJ, Dimaggio C, Karpati A. Estimated deaths attributable to social factors in the United States. Am J Publ Health. 2011;101(8):1456–65.
7. Hahn RA. Racial and ethnic residential segregation as a root social determinant of public health and health inequity: a persistent public health challenge in the United States. Poverty Race. 2017;26(2):3–4; 10-15.
8. The Burden of Disease Collaborators, Mokdad AH, Ballestros K, Echko M, Glenn S, Olsen HE, Mullany E, et al. The state of US health, 1990-2016: Burden of diseases, injuries, and risk factors among US states. JAMA. 2018;319(14):1444–72.
9. Daniel H, Bornstein SS, Kane GC, Health and Public Policy Committee of the American College of Physicians. Addressing social determinants to improve patient care and promote health equity: an American College of Physicians Position Paper. Ann Intern Med. 2018;168(8):577–8.
10. Diez Roux AV, Mair C. Neighborhoods and health. Ann N Y Acad Sci. 2010;1186:125–45.
11. Diez Roux AV, Merkin SS, Arnet D, Chambliss L, Massing M, Nieto FJ, et al. Neighborhood of residence and incidence of coronary heart disease. N Engl J Med. 2001;345(2):99–106.
12. Brown AF, Liang LJ, Vasser SD, Merkin SS, Longstreth WT Jr, Ovbiagele B, et al. Neighborhood socioeconomic disadvantage and mortality after stroke. Neurology. 2013;80(6):520–7.

13. Bikdeli B, Wayda B, Bao H, Riss JS, Xu X, Chaudry SI, et al. Place of residence and outcomes of patients with heart failure: analysis from the telemonitoring to improve heart failure outcomes trial. Circ Cardiovasc Qual Outcomes. 2014;7(5):749–56.
14. Agarwal S, Garg A, Parashar A, Jaber WA, Menon V. Outcomes and resource utilization in ST-elevation myocardial infarction in the United States: evidence for socioeconomic disparities. J Am Heart Assoc. 2014;3(6):e001057.
15. Levine RS, Foster JE, Fullilove RE, Fullilove MT, Briggs NC, Hull PC, et al. Black-white inequalities in mortality and life expectancy, 1933-1999: implications for healthy people 2010. Public Health Rep. 2001;116(5):474–83.
16. Heidenreich PA, Albert NM, Allen LA, Bluemke DA, Butler J, Fonarow GC, et al. Forecasting the impact of heart failure in the United States. Circ Heart Fail. 2013;6(3):606–19.
17. Morris AA, McAllister P, Grant A, Geng S, Kelli HM, Kalogeropoulos A, et al. Relation of living in a "food desert" to recurrent hospitalizations in patients with heart failure. Am J Cardiol. 2019;123(2):291–6.
18. Robert SA. Community-level socioeconomic status effects on adult health. J Health Soc Behav. 1998;39(1):18–37.
19. Michalsen A, König G, Thimme W. Preventable causative factors leading to hospital admission with decompensated heart failure. Heart. 1998;80(5):437–41.
20. Walker RE, Keane CR, Burke JG. Disparities and access to healthy foods in the United States: a review of food deserts literature. Health Place. 2010;16(5):876–84.
21. Koh HK, Parekh AK. Toward a United States of health: implications of understanding the US burden of disease. JAMA. 2018;319(14):1438–40.
22. Koh HK. Improving health and health care in the United States—toward a state of complete well-being. JAMA. 2016;316(16):1679–81.
23. Dieleman JL, Baral R, Birger M, Bui AL, Bulchis A, Chapin A, et al. US spending on healthcare and public health, 1996-2013. JAMA. 2016;316(24):2627–46.
24. Bradley EH, Taylor LA. The American paradox: why spending more is getting us less. Philadelphia: Public Affairs Books; 2013.
25. Koh HK, Rajkumar R, McDonough JE. Reframing prevention in the era of health reform. JAMA. 2016;316(10):1039–40.
26. Woolf SH, Aron L, editors. U.S. health in international perspective: shorter lives, poorer health. Washington, DC: National Academies Press; 2013.
27. Annas GJ, Galea S. Dying healthy: public health priorities for fixed population life expectancies. Ann Intern Med. 2018;169(8):568–9.
28. Adler NE, Newman K. Socioeconomic disparities in health: pathways and policies. Health Aff (Millwood). 2002;21(2):60–76.
29. Diez Roux AV. Investigating neighborhood and area effects on health. Am J Public Health. 2001;91(11):1783–9.
30. Naryan KMV, Patel SA, Cunningham SA, Curran J. Ominous reversal of health gains in the United States: time to rethink research priorities? Ann Intern Med. 2019;170(5):330–1.
31. Link BG, Phelan J. Social conditions as fundamental causes of disease. J Health Soc Behav. 1995;Spec No:80–94.
32. Ludwig J, Sanbonmatsu L, Gennetian L, Adam E, Duncan GJ, Katz LF, et al. Neighborhoods, obesity, and diabetes-a randomized social experiment. N Engl J Med. 2011;365(16):1509–19.
33. Kind AJ, Jencks S, Brock J, Yu M, Bartels C, Ehlenbach W, et al. Neighborhood socioeconomic disadvantage and 30-day rehospitalization: a retrospective cohort study. Ann Intern Med. 2014;161(11):765–74.
34. Kind AJH, Buckingham WR. Making neighborhood-disadvantage metrics accessible -t he neighborhood atlas. N Engl J Med. 2018;378(26):2456–8.

Conclusion and Afterword

10

Introduction

The book that you have just read contains a great deal of medical, socioeconomic, demographic, epidemiologic, racial, ethnic, educational, and cultural information pertaining particularly to the black population of the United States, but it is admittedly somewhat incomplete. There is so much more that might have been included, but space and time limitations preclude a more comprehensive coverage of everything that touches upon the healthcare scene involving black Americans. In this brief postscript, I would like to suggest to the reader to consider a few more important issues affecting black health.

Additional Healthcare Issues Affecting the Black Community

Low Recruitment of Black Students into Medical Careers

The problem of insufficient recruitment of African American students into careers in medicine is often referred to as the medical school "pipeline" problem, which has been highlighted by several incisive publications such as *An American Crisis: The Growing Absence of Black Men in Medicine and Science*, a book whose lead author was Cato T. Laurencin, MD, PhD, Rapporteur for the National Academies of Sciences, Engineering, and Medicine [1]. In the Proceedings of a Joint Workshop in which several prominent luminaries participated, it was pointed out that blacks, and black men in particular, are underrepresented among medical school applicants (Fig. 10.1) [2]. As Louis Sullivan, MD, Chairman and CEO of the Sullivan Alliance to Transform the Health Professions, noted in his keynote speech, although African Americans constitute 13% of the US population, they constitute only 7% of medical students and less than 3% of practicing doctors. In addition, we seem to be reversing course regarding the admission of black men to medical school; in 1978, 542 black males matriculated in medical schools compared to 515 blacks in 2014

© Springer Nature Switzerland AG 2020
R. A. Williams, *Blacks in Medicine*, https://doi.org/10.1007/978-3-030-41960-8_10

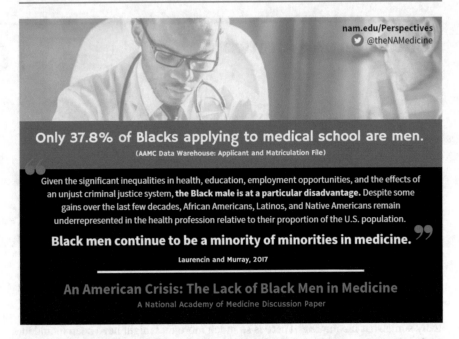

Fig. 10.1 Black males are not applying to medical schools in sufficient numbers. (Data from Laurencin and Murray [2]; graphic courtesy of the National Academy of Medicine https://nam.edu/an-american-crisis-the-lack-of-black-men-in-medicine/)

(Fig. 10.2) [2]. Thus, the pipeline has grown narrower, with insufficient numbers of black doctors eventually being produced. This has ramifications for the black community, since it has been shown that black patients elect to receive more preventive care when the providers are black as compared to when they are not [3]. In addition, physicians who are members of underrepresented groups are more likely than whites to serve poor, minority, and Medicaid populations [4]. There is also a need for more diversity in leadership positions in academic medicine. As stated by Cantor et al., "diversity improves patient care….promoting women and underrepresented minorities to leadership positions may well enable academic medicine to better serve our diverse population" [5]. Only 2% of full-time medical school faculty consists of black men, according to the Association of American Medical Colleges (AAMC).

Violence in the Black Community

Violence in the black community is a problem that has flown under the radar until recently, when the National Medical Association (NMA) created a task force to address it. The *NMA's Working Group on Gun Violence and Police Use of Force*, of which I was a member, was led by national co-chairs Roger A. Mitchell, Jr., MD, Chief Medical Examiner for the District of Columbia, and

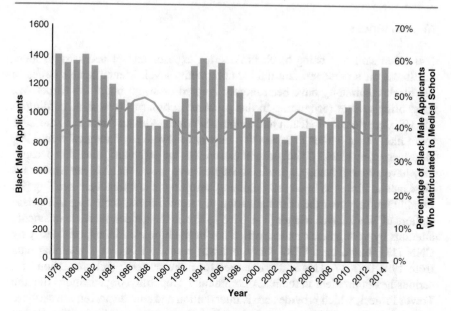

Fig. 10.2 Number of black or African American male medical school applicants (bars) versus percentage of black or African American applicants who matriculated (line), 1978–2014. Source: AAMC Data Warehouse: Applicant and Matriculant File, as of 5/11/2015. (From Laurencin and Murray [2] with permission Springer)

Eva Louise Frazer, MD, an internist and prominent community activist from St. Louis, Missouri [6]. Following an initial White Paper on the subject, a full-scale article was published and disseminated in 2018 [7]. The report detailed the police use of excessive force, and many approaches to reducing the level of violence were suggested, including greater involvement by the community of black physicians who must play a vital role in eradicating this epidemic. More interaction between the police, physicians, and the public was recommended.

The NMA has begun discussions with the National Organization of Black Law Enforcement Executives (NOBLE; https://noblenational.org/) on the issue of violence and the police use of force in the black community. This dialogue has been facilitated by former Norfolk, Virginia, Chief of Police and former NOBLE President John I. Dixon III and Sheila L. Thorne, President and CEO of the Multicultural Healthcare Marketing Group, who have collaborated with the NMA and other medical groups in communities of color to develop strategies to combat this problem, which is spreading explosively throughout the country.

Recently, there has been speculation that exposure to violence has had psycho-pathological fallout in the black community with the development of post-traumatic stress disorder (PTSD), which is defined as a trauma- or stress-related reaction that may develop in individuals following exposure to an ordeal or an event in which death or physical harm has occurred, is witnessed, or is threatened. This is another example of the public health consequences of violence and police brutality in the black community, leading to a population that may be in need of psychotherapy.

Mental Illness

It is often said that being black in America exposes one of necessity to mental illness on a personal, familial, or community level. Mental health issues in the black community have been largely ignored or swept under the carpet. We must bring greater recognition to this problem in order to treat it. According to the US Department of Health and Human Services, African Americans are 20% more likely than whites to report that they have severe psychological stress [8]. However, many blacks do not present themselves for psychiatric attention because they have a fear of being stigmatized; studies have shown that African Americans view mental illness as highly stigmatizing, resulting in low treatment-seeking [9]. In addition, they fear the criminalization of mental illness, according to Patrisse Cullors of Black Lives Matter [10]. Tied to this is the sudden increase in suicide attempts by young black males, which has been chronicled in a special story by CNN [11], based on a CDC study that was recently released, containing data from 1991 to 2017. This is a prime area for more research and prevention of a serious health problem in the black community. Hopefully, organizations like the Trevor Project, which provides crisis intervention and suicide prevention services primarily to LGBTQ/Q young people, will become more involved in the special situation facing black youth, who are more impacted by poverty, low income, joblessness, racism, and homelessness.

High Maternal Mortality

High maternal mortality is a problem that the black community has silently dealt with for decades. It has several definitions. One definition is death of a woman while pregnant or within 42 days of end of pregnancy, irrespective of the cause of death. Defined as the number of maternal or pregnancy-related deaths in a given time period per 100,000 live births during the same period, the maternal mortality rate has been rising for American women in general but much more so for black women, who experience more than three times the rate that white women do. In fact, as Fig. 10.3 shows, the statistics for black women in the United States are closer to women from Brazil, Uzbekistan, Malaysia, and Mexico compared to non-Hispanic American white women whose statistical profile resembles that of women in more affluent countries such as Japan, New Zealand, the United Kingdom, and France [12]. There is also a difference in causation of pregnancy-related deaths between blacks and whites, as reported by a study of Maternal Mortality Review Committee data by the Building US Capacity to Review and Prevent Maternal Deaths initiative, a partnership of the Association of Maternal and Child Health Programs (AMCHP), the Centers for Disease Control and Prevention (CDC) Division of Reproductive Health, and CDC Foundation (Fig. 10.4) [13]. The main causes in blacks are cardiomyopathy, preeclampsia, and eclampsia, whereas the principal causes in whites are cardiovascular and coronary conditions, hemorrhage, mental health conditions, and infections.

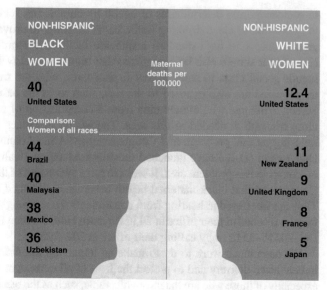

MORTALITY GAP FOR U.S. MOMS

In the U.S., black women who are expecting or who are new mothers died at rates similar to those of the same women in lower-income countries, while the maternal mortality rate for white U.S. mothers more closely resembles rates in more affluent nations.

NON-HISPANIC BLACK WOMEN

Maternal deaths per 100,000

NON-HISPANIC WHITE WOMEN

40
United States

12.4
United States

Comparison:
Women of all races

44
Brazil

11
New Zealand

40
Malaysia

9
United Kingdom

38
Mexico

8
France

36
Uzbekistan

5
Japan

Source: U.S. ratios (2011-2014): CDC Pregnancy Mortality Surveillance System; Global ratios (2015): UNICEF

Fig. 10.3 The mortality gap between non-Hispanic black and white women in the United States and comparison with selected countries of the world. (From Roeder [12], with permission. Illustration courtesy of Ben S. Wallace, Harvard T.H. Chan School of Public Health)

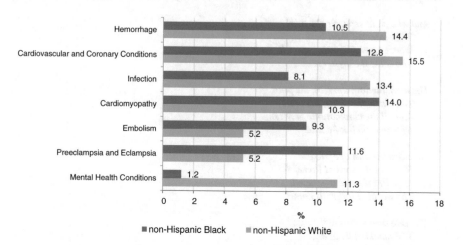

Fig. 10.4 Building US Capacity to Review and Prevent Maternal Deaths. (2018). Report from nine maternal mortality review committees. (Retrieved from http://reviewtoaction.org/Report_from_Nine_MMRCs. Accessed 6 Nov 2019)

Members of the Congressional Black Caucus, and Senator Kamala Harris in particular, have expressed grave concern about these disparities in maternal mortality. Senator Harris says that racial bias is part of the cause. Senator Elizabeth Warren agrees. One area of focus is on prevention; it is estimated that about two-thirds of black maternal deaths are entirely preventable if more attention is paid to socioeconomic determinants of health by eliminating social inequities through the provision of clean drinking water, better housing, improved transportation, and greater access to high-standard healthcare facilities for pre- and postnatal care. However, it should also be recognized that higher mortality in black women transcends social class to some extent in that those who are more affluent and better educated are also exposed to the risk, such as in the case of black tennis star Serena Williams, who almost died from a complication of pregnancy. Obviously, more research is needed in this area. The March of Dimes is one agency that is focusing on this problem, and Congresswomen Alma Adams (D-NC) and Lauren Underwood (D-IL) have launched the Black Maternal Health Caucus to improve outcomes in this problem area. It seeks to raise awareness of the condition in the US Congress so that black maternal health becomes established as a national priority. They are interested in hearing from constituents from throughout the country. They may be reached at their office at 2436 Rayburn House Office Building, Washington, DC, 20515–3312 or by calling their office at 202–225-1510.

We have much work to do to make an impact on the factors causing disparities in healthcare delivery and to protect the lives of all citizens of the United States, and especially of those who are the most vulnerable, such as the black population and other people of color. It is my hope that one day it will be unnecessary to make efforts like this on behalf of discrete segments of our society, because we will all truly be equal. The poem *Common Dust* by black poet Georgia Douglas Johnson expresses that hope:

> *And who shall separate the dust.*
> *What later we shall be:*
> *Whose keen discerning eye will scan.*
> *And solve the mystery?*

> *The high, the low, the rich, the poor,*
> *The black, the white, the red,*
> *And all the chromatique between,*
> *Of whom shall it be said:*

> *Here lies the dust of Africa;*
> *Here are the sons of Rome;*
> *Here lies the one unlabeled,*
> *The world at large his home!*

> *Can one then separate the dust?*
> *Will mankind lie apart,*
> *When life has settled back again.*
> *The same as from the start?*

As this book was going into production, evidence of a growing awareness of the racial, ethnic, and cultural divide and the importance of recognizing our historical legacy emerged in a photograph that circulated virally on social media and news organizations, showing 15 African American medical students from Tulane University in New Orleans standing in front of the former slave quarters of the Whitney Plantation in Wallace, Louisiana, about 46 miles northwest of New Orleans, on December 14, 2019 (students listed alphabetically: Tivona Batieste, Christen Brown, Carrie Crook, Mashli Fleurestil, Adedoyin Johnson, Alexandria Jones, Sydney Labat, Jean Lafontant, Russell J. Ledet, Jessica Mecklosky, Tiana Roddy, Jasmine Taylor, Rachel

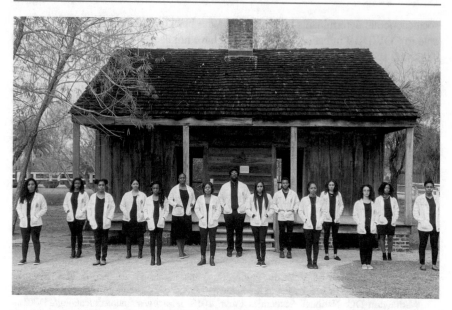

Fig. 10.5 African American medical students from Tulane University in New Orleans standing in front of a former slave quarters of the Whitney Plantation in Wallace, Louisiana, about 46 miles northwest of New Orleans, on December 14, 2019. "We are our ancestors' wildest dreams," student Russell J. Ledet wrote in a tweet sharing a photograph of the moment. (Photograph courtesy of Brian Washington Jr., with permission)

Trusty, Rachel Turner, Jasira Ziglar). "We are our ancestors' wildest dreams," student Russell J. Ledet wrote in a tweet sharing a photograph of the moment (Fig. 10.5). Thus, our saga of Blacks in Medicine has come full circle, from the shackles of slavery to the halls of sophisticated medical schools, and back, to revisit the place where so much suffering occurred. We can thank those students for providing the connection between the brutal past and the bright future that awaits them.

Also, as this book was about to go to press, the coronavirus (COVID-19) pandemic erupted and is still largely uncontrolled at the time of this writing. Although it is not possible to review all aspects of this crisis in this small space, it is important to mention some relevant issues regarding the disproportionate impact that this disease is having on communities of color in the United States. Early data indicates that the occurrence rate and the death rate are disproportionately high in large cities even where African Americans are not the majority of the population. For instance, according to CNN host and journalist Van Jones, who spoke on CNN on April 6, 2020 in an opinion piece titled "Black America Must Wake Up to this Viral Threat", in Milwaukee County, Wisconsin, where 27 percent of the residents are black, almost half of those infected with the virus are black, and 81 percent of those who died of COVID-19 are African American. In Illinois, where blacks make up only 14.6 percent of the population, 28 percent of those affected are black. In Michigan, including Detroit, blacks account for 33 percent of the cases and 40 percent of the deaths. And in Louisiana, where blacks are not in the majority, Governor John Bel Edwards has indicated that almost 70 percent of the deaths are in black people. Why is this happening? One might speculate that the co-morbidities that predominate in black communities such as high rates of heart disease, hypertension, diabetes, asthma, cancer, and other disorders, combined with a high incidence of the socioeconomic determinants of health make the black population particularly vulnerable to COVID-19 infection. All of the data have not been gathered because very few cities and states are tracking the incidence and deaths by race and ethnicity, which is necessary to draw a clear picture of what is going on. Without that data, resources and funding such as money from the recently passed $2 trillion dollar Stimulus bill may not be appropriately distributed to those in poor communities of color where the need for relief seems to be the greatest. And more information and data should be demanded from the Centers for Disease Control and Prevention (CDC) which so far has been reluctant to release anything to the public, despite requests made by some congressmen including Senator Wyden of Oregon. We can and must do more to avert unnecessary deaths and suffering from this deadly scourge. Blacks, including African American organizations, must come to the rescue of themselves before it is too late.

References

1. National Academies of Sciences, Engineering, and Medicine. An American Crisis: The Growing Absence of Black Men in Medicine and Science: Proceedings of a Joint Workshop. Washington DC: National Academies Press. 2018. https://www.nap.edu/catalog/25130/an-american-crisis-the-growing-absence-of-black-men-in. Accessed 30 Oct 2019.
2. Laurencin CT, Murray M. An American crisis: the lack of black men in medicine. J Racial Ethnic Health Disparities. 2017;4:317–21.
3. Alsan M, Garrick O, Graziani GC. Does diversity matter for health? Experimental evidence from Oakland. NBER Working Paper No. 24787. Issued Jun 2018, Revised Aug 2019. Cambridge, MA: National Bureau of Economic Research, 2018. https://www.nber.org/papers/w24787. Accessed 30 Oct 2019.
4. Cantor JC, Miles EL, Baker LC, Barker DC. Physician service to the underserved: implications for affirmative action in medical education. Inquiry. 1996;33(2):167–80.
5. Beeler WH, Mangurian C, Jagsi R. Unplugging the pipeline – a call for term limits in academic medicine. N Engl J Med. 2019;381(16):1508–11.
6. Jones A. National Medical Association seeks to address violence in the African American community. Philadelphia Tribune. 2 Aug 2017. https://www.nmanet.org/news/359921/NMA-seeks-to-address-violence-in-the-African-American-community.htm. Accessed 30 Dec 2019.
7. Frazer E, Mitchell RA, Nesbitt LS, Williams M, Mitchell EP, Williams RA, Browne D. The violence epidemic in the African American community: a call by the National Medical Association for comprehensive reform. J Nat Med Assoc. 2018;110(1):4–15.
8. Mental Health America. Black & African American communities and mental health. https://www.mhanational.org/issues/black-african-american-communities-and-mental-health. Accessed 30 Oct 2019.
9. Ward EC, Wiltshire JC, Detry MA, Brown RL. African American men and women's attitude toward mental illness, perceptions of stigma, and preferred coping behaviors. Nurs Res. 2013;62(3):185–94.
10. Black Lives Matter's Patrice Cullors on the criminalization of mental illness. https://www.mic.com/. 11 Oct 2019. https://www.mic.com/p/black-lives-matters-patrisse-cullors-on-the-criminalization-of-mental-illness-19209822. Accessed 30 Oct 2019.
11. Christensen J. Suicide attempts by black teens are increasing, study says. https://www.cnn.com/2019/10/14/health/black-teen-suicide-attempts-study/index.html. Accessed 30 Oct 2019.
12. Roeder A. America is failing its black mothers. Harvard Public Health. Winter 2019. https://www.hsph.harvard.edu/magazine/magazine_article/america-is-failing-its-black-mothers/. Accessed 30 Oct 2019.
13. Review to Action. Building U.S. capacity to review and prevent maternal deaths. Report from nine maternal mortality review committees. https://reviewtoaction.org/Report_from_Nine_MMRCs. Accessed 21 Oct 2019.

Index

© Springer Nature Switzerland AG 2020
R. A. Williams, *Blacks in Medicine*, https://doi.org/10.1007/978-3-030-41960-8

Printed in the United States
by Baker & Taylor Publisher Services